Pancreaticobiliary and Luminal Stents

Guest Editor

TODD H. BARON, MD

GASTROINTESTINAL ENDOSCOPY CLINICS OF NORTH AMERICA

www.giendo.theclinics.com

Consulting Editor
CHARLES J. LIGHTDALE, MD

July 2011 • Volume 21 • Number 3

SAUNDERS an imprint of ELSEVIER, Inc.

W.B. SAUNDERS COMPANY
A Division of Elsevier Inc.

1600 John F. Kennedy Blvd. ● Suite 1800 ● Philadelphia, Pennsylvania 19103-2899

http://www.giendo.theclinics.com

GASTROINTESTINAL ENDOSCOPY CLINICS OF NORTH AMERICA Volume 21, Number 3
July 2011 ISSN 1052-5157, ISBN-13: 978-1-4557-1098-0

Editor: Kerry Holland
Developmental Editor: Donald Mumford

Gastrointestinal Endoscopy Clinics of North America (ISSN 1052-5157) is published quarterly by Elsevier Inc., 360 Park Avenue South, New York, NY 10010-1710. Months of issue are January, April, July, and October. Business and Editorial Offices: 1600 John F. Kennedy Blvd., Suite 1800, Philadelphia, PA, 19103-2899. Periodicals postage paid at New York, NY and additional mailing offices. Subscription prices are $295.00 per year for US individuals, $414.00 per year for US institutions, $156.00 per year for US students and residents, $325.00 per year for Canadian individuals, $505.00 per year for Canadian institutions, $412.00 per year for international individuals, $505.00 per year for international institutions, and $217.00 per year for Canadian and foreign students/residents. To receive student/resident rate, orders must be accompanied by name of affiliated institution, date of term, and the *signature* of program/residency coordinator on institution letterhead. Orders will be billed at individual rate until proof of status is received. Foreign air speed delivery is included in all *Clinics* subscription prices. All prices are subject to change without notice. **POSTMASTER:** Send address change to *Gastrointestinal Endoscopy Clinics of North America*, Elsevier Health Sciences Division, Subscription Customer Service, 3251 Riverport Lane, Maryland Heights, MO 63043. **Customer Service: 1-800-654-2452 (US). From outside the United States, call 1-314-447-8871. Fax: 1-314-447-8029. E-mail: JournalsCustomerService-usa@elsevier.com (for print support) or JournalsOnlineSupport-usa@elsevier.com (for online support).**

Reprints. For copies of 100 or more, of articles in this publication, please contact the Commercial Reprints Department, Elsevier Inc., 360 Park Avenue South, New York, NY 10010-1710. Tel. (212) 633-3812; Fax: (212) 482-1935; E-mail: reprints@elsevier.com.

Gastrointestinal Endoscopy Clinics of North America is covered in *Excerpta Medica, MEDLINE/PubMed (Index Medicus), and MEDLINE/MEDLARS.*

Contributors

CONSULTING EDITOR

CHARLES J. LIGHTDALE, MD
Professor, Department of Medicine, Columbia University Medical Center, New York, New York

GUEST EDITOR

TODD H. BARON, MD, FASGE
Professor of Medicine, Division of Gastroenterology and Hepatology, Department of Medicine, Mayo Clinic, Rochester, Minnesota

AUTHORS

DOUGLAS G. ADLER, MD, FACG, AGAF, FASGE
Associate Professor of Medicine; Director of Therapeutic Endoscopy, Gastroenterology and Hepatology, University of Utah School of Medicine, Salt Lake City, Utah

MIHIR R. BAKHRU, MD, MSc
Division of Gastroenterology and Hepatology, University of Virginia Health System, Charlottesville, Virginia

IVO BOSKOSKI, MD
Digestive Endoscopy Unit, Gemelli University Hospital, Universita' Cattolica del Sacro Cuore, Roma, Italy

BRYAN BRIMHALL, MD
Division of Gastroenterology and Hepatology, Department of Internal Medicine, University of Utah School of Medicine, Salt Lake City, Utah

GUIDO COSTAMAGNA, MD, FACG
Digestive Endoscopy Unit, Gemelli University Hospital, Universita' Cattolica del Sacro Cuore, Roma, Italy

JACQUES DEVIERE, MD, PhD
Professor of Medicine, Chairman, Department of Gastroenterology, Hepatopancreatology and Digestive Oncology, Erasme University Hospital, Université Libre de Bruxelles, Brussels, Belgium

KULWINDER S. DUA, MD, FACP, FRCP (Edinburgh), FRCP (London), FASGE
Professor, Division of Gastroenterology and Hepatology, Department of Medicine; Director, Advanced Endoscopy Training Program, Medical College of Wisconsin, Milwaukee, Wisconsin

PIETRO FAMILIARI, MD, PhD
Digestive Endoscopy Unit, Gemelli University Hospital, Universita' Cattolica del Sacro Cuore, Roma, Italy

DANIEL DE PAULA PESSOA FERREIRA, MD
Fellow of the Digestive Endoscopy Unit, IRCCS Istituto Clinico Humanitas, Milan, Italy

PAUL FOCKENS, MD, PhD
Professor and Chairman, Department of Gastroenterology and Hepatology, Academic Medical Center, University of Amsterdam, Amsterdam, The Netherlands

CHRISTIAN GERGES, MD
Department of Internal Medicine, Evangelisches Krankenhaus Düsseldorf, Duesseldorf, Germany

INGE HUIBREGTSE, MD, PhD
Fellow in Gastroenterology and Hepatology, Department of Gastroenterology and Hepatology, Academic Medical Center, University of Amsterdam, Amsterdam, The Netherlands

MICHEL KAHALEH, MD
Division of Gastroenterology and Hepatology; Associate Professor of Medicine, Director, Pancreatico-Biliary Services, Division of Gastroenterology and Hepatology, University of Virginia Health System, Charlottesville, Virginia

RICHARD A. KOZAREK, MD
Digestive Disease Institute, Virginia Mason Medical Center, Seattle, Washington

JEFFREY H. LEE, MD, FACG, FASGE
Professor and Director, Advanced Endoscopy Fellowship, Department of Gastroenterology, Hepatology, and Nutrition, MD Anderson Cancer Center, Houston, Texas

HORST NEUHAUS, MD
Department of Internal Medicine, Evangelisches Krankenhaus Düsseldorf, Düsseldorf, Germany

VINCENZO PERRI, MD
Digestive Endoscopy Unit, Gemelli University Hospital, Universita' Cattolica del Sacro Cuore, Roma, Italy

ALESSANDRO REPICI, MD
Director of the Digestive Endoscopy Unit, IRCCS Istituto Clinico Humanitas, Milan, Italy

ANDREW S. ROSS, MD
Digestive Disease Institute, Virginia Mason Medical Center, Seattle, Washington

BRIGITTE SCHUMACHER, MD
Department of Internal Medicine, Evangelisches Krankenhaus Düsseldorf, Düsseldorf, Germany

P.D. SIERSEMA, MD, PhD, FASGE, FACG
Professor of Gastroenterology and Hepatology, Head, Department of Gastroenterology and Hepatology, University Medical Center Utrecht, Utrecht, The Netherlands

GRISCHA TERHEGGEN, MD
Department of Internal Medicine, Evangelisches Krankenhaus Düsseldorf, Düsseldorf, Germany

ANDREA TRINGALI, MD, PhD
Digestive Endoscopy Unit, Gemelli University Hospital, Universita' Cattolica del Sacro
Cuore, Roma, Italy

NIMISH VAKIL, MD, FACP, FACG, AGAF
Professor of Medicine, Department of Gastroenterology, Aurora Summit Hospital,
University of Wisconsin School of Medicine and Public Health, Madison, Wisconsin

F.P. VLEGGAAR, MD, PhD
Associate Professor of Gastroenterology and Hepatology, Chief of Endoscopy,
Department of Gastroenterology and Hepatology, University Medical Center Utrecht,
Utrecht, The Netherlands

Contents

> Expandable stents are widely used in gastroenterology. The basic princi-
> ple of all of these devices is that they can be constrained onto a delivery
> system of small diameter and then deployed in an area of stenosis without
> the risk of complications due to excessive dilation. Understanding tissue
> responses to stents is important both for the design of new stents and
> for clinicians to balance the benefits and risks of covered and uncovered
> stents. With biodegradable stents and removable stents, understanding
> tissue responses provides the basis for timing of removal and assessing
> treatment response.

> Partially covered self-expandable esophageal stents have been associ-
> ated with unacceptable complications when used for benign esophageal
> disorders. With the introduction of removable or potentially removable fully
> covered stents and biodegradable stents, interest in using expandable
> stents for benign indications has been revived. Although expandable
> stents can offer a minimally invasive alternative to surgery, they can be as-
> sociated with serious complications; hence, this approach should be
> considered in carefully selected patients, preferably on a protocol basis.

> Esophageal cancer is diagnosed in about 400,000 patients each year
> worldwide, and its incidence is increasing faster than that of any other ma-
> lignancy. This makes it the ninth most common malignancy and sixth on
> the list of cancer mortality causes. Most patients with esophageal cancer
> present at a stage that is too advanced for curative therapy, and many die
> within a few months. Treatment of dysphagia is the main goal of palliative
> care in more than 50% of incurable cases. Although many different pallia-
> tive options for malignant dysphagia are available, expandable stent
> placement is the most commonly performed treatment modality.

> Malignant gastric outlet obstruction (GOO) is a commonly encountered en-
> tity, defined as the inability of the stomach to empty because of

mechanical obstruction at the level of either the stomach or the proximal small bowel. In this article, current literature on GOO is reviewed with a focus on enteral stents to include symptoms and diagnosis, stent and non-stent treatment, types of enteral stents, indications and contraindications to stent placement, and technical and clinical success rates. In comparison with gastrojejunostomy, enteral stent placement is better suited for patients with a shorter life expectancy and/or those who are poor surgical candidates.

Vincenzo Perri, Pietro Familiari, Andrea Tringali, Ivo Boskoski, and Guido Costamagna

Biliary plastic stenting plays a key role in the endoscopic management of benign biliary diseases. Complications following surgery of the biliary tract and liver transplantation are amenable to endoscopic treatment by plastic stenting. Insertion of an increasing number of plastic stents is currently the method of choice to treat postoperative biliary strictures. Benign biliary strictures secondary to chronic pancreatitis or primary sclerosing cholangitis may benefit from plastic stenting in select cases. There is a role for plastic stent placement in nonoperative candidates with acute cholecystitis and in patients with irretrievable bile duct stones.

Inge Huibregtse and Paul Fockens

Plastic biliary endoprostheses have not changed much since their introduction more than 3 decades ago. Although their use has been challenged by the introduction of metal stents, plastic stents still remain commonly used. Much work has been done to improve the problem of stent obstruction but without substantial clinical success. In this review, the authors discuss the history of plastic biliary stent development and the current use of plastic stents for malignant biliary diseases.

Mihir R. Bakhru and Michel Kahaleh

Benign biliary diseases include benign biliary strictures (BBS), choledocholithiasis, and leaks. BBS encompass postoperative injury, anastomotic stricture, chronic pancreatitis, primary sclerosing cholangitis, and gallstone-related stricture. Therapeutic options for benign biliary diseases include surgical, percutaneous, and endoscopic interventions. Endoscopic options include placement of plastic stents as well as self-expanding metal stents (SEMS). SEMS can be uncovered, partially covered, and fully covered, and have been used with some success in resolution of strictures and leaks; however, complications limit their use. This article reviews the currently published experience on SEMS and attempts to define their current role in the treatment of benign biliary diseases.

Jeffrey H. Lee

Obstructive jaundice can result from benign or malignant etiologies. The common benign conditions include primary sclerosing cholangitis, chronic pancreatitis, and gallstones. Malignant biliary obstruction can be caused by direct tumor infiltration, extrinsic compression by enlarged lymph nodes or malignant lesions, adjacent inflammation, desmoplastic reaction from a tumor, or a combination of these factors. Malignant diseases causing biliary obstruction include pancreatic cancer, ampullary cancer, cholangiocarcinoma, and metastatic diseases. This article focuses on malignant distal biliary obstruction and its management.

Most patients with malignant hilar stenoses are candidates for palliation. For this purpose, biliary drainage plays a major role in improving liver function and managing or avoiding cholangitis. Endoscopic interventions are less invasive than the percutaneous approach and should be considered as the first-line drainage procedures in most cases. Transhepatic interventions should be reserved for endoscopic failures or performed as a complementary approach in a combined procedure. After successful endoscopic access to biliary obstruction, implantation of self-expandable metal stents offers advantages over plastic endoprostheses in terms of stent patency and number of reinterventions.

Use of stents in the pancreas has been confined and limited to referral centers that specialize in the treatment of patients with severe pancreatitis and acute relapsing pancreatitis. With therapeutic development in endoscopic treatment of pancreatic diseases and a better understanding of the cause and prevention of ERCP related complications, the use of stents has been extended to transmural drainage of pancreatic fluid collection or of pancreatic ducts has well as to prophylaxis of post-ERCP pancreatitis. As a result, indication for pancreatic stenting and the kind of stents to be used as well as the followup after placement varies. This article reviews the major indication for pancreatic stent placement and focuses on the choice of stent, technique of implantation and followup.

The surgical management of malignant colorectal obstruction is still controversial and has higher associated mortality and complication rates compared with elective surgery. Placement of self-expanding metallic stents (SEMS) has been proposed as an alternative therapeutic approach for colonic decompression of patients with acute malignant obstruction. SEMS placement may be used both as a bridge to surgery in patients who are good candidates for curative resection and for palliation of those patients presenting with advanced stage disease or with severe comorbid medical illnesses.

The use of stents throughout the gastrointestinal tract has evolved over the past century. The evolution of endoscopic ultrasound and significant improvements in stent design are key factors that have allowed endoscopists to drive the use of stents in gastroenterology into new directions. Endoscopic creativity remains crucial in the evolution of any new endoscopic technology. Finally, the use of multidisciplinary teams, including endoscopists, radiologists, and surgeons, allows for the exchange of ideas and procedural planning necessary for successful innovation.

THE CLINICS ARE NOW AVAILABLE ONLINE!

Access your subscription at:
www.theclinics.com

Foreword

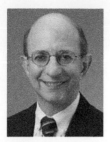

Charles J. Lightdale, MD
Consulting Editor

Placing stents to maintain patency of ducts and lumens has become a major thera-peutic tool for interventional gastrointestinal endoscopists. The evolution from hand-made rigid stents to a wide array of flexible, expandable metal and plastic devices has been rapid and remarkable. GI stents provide successful treatment, and palliation for an extensive variety of blockages, obstructions, and stenoses within the esoph-agus, stomach, small intestine, and colon, have become staples in interventional ERCP and are key elements in the developing field of therapeutic EUS. GI stents will no doubt continue to proliferate and improve, driven in no small part by the enormous markets for stents in cardiology and interventional radiology.

With the increasing use of GI stents, and the availability of multiple novel devices requiring selection decisions, and new endoscopic techniques and skills, it seemed timely to devote an issue of the *Gastrointestinal Endoscopy Clinics of North America* to "Pancreatobiliary and Gastrointestinal Stents." I am delighted that Todd Baron, a leader in the field, is the guest editor for this volume. He has gathered an extraordi-nary group of expert authors on topics in GI stenting and has crafted a splendid issue of the *Clinics*. Just like a stent, this issue affords an "opening" that should interest everyone in gastrointestinal endoscopy.

Charles J. Lightdale, MD
Department of Medicine
Columbia University Medical Center
161 Fort Washington Avenue, Room 812
New York, NY 10032, USA

E-mail address:
CJL18@columbia.edu

Gastrointest Endoscopy Clin N Am 21 (2011) xiii
doi:10.1016/j.giec.2011.04.014
1052-5157/11/$ – see front matter © 2011 Elsevier Inc. All rights reserved.

Preface

Pancreaticobiliary and Gastrointestinal Stents

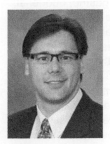

Todd H. Baron, MD
Guest Editor

When searching PubMed, the term "stent" first appeared in the title of a publication in 1952. At the time of this writing, a search in PubMed using "stent" produced 52,629 articles. The origin has been conjectured to be from the Scottish word stynt or stent, meaning stretched out river fishing nets (an extension if you will). However, in an excellent review by Sterioff on the etymology of the word stent,[1] it is widely accepted that the word evolved from Stent's compound, created by British dentist Charles. T. Stent (1807–1885) and used for dental impressions. Subsequently, in 1917 a surgeon, Johannes F.S. Esser (1877–1946), used the compound for facial plastic surgery and referred to it as Stent's mould.[2] In 1954, William H. Re Mine and John H. Grindlay used Stent's principle to create omentum-lined plastic tubes in the reconstruction of canine bile ducts[3]; surgically placed biliary tubes (stents) were quickly adopted. In 1974 Molnar and Stockum were the first to describe percutaneous placement of a plastic biliary stent[4] and in 1979 Soehendra and Reynders-Frederix described endoscopic placement for palliation of malignant biliary obstruction.[5] Development of expandable metal stents for endoscopic use lagged behind cardiology and interventional radiology use, and expandable metal stents were first developed for palliation of malignant biliary and esophageal obstruction followed by stents developed for palliation of gastroduodenal and colonic obstruction. It is remarkable that endoscopic gastrointestinal stent technology (stents passed through endoscopes) is relatively recent, with expandable metal stents first used within the last 20 years.

At the present time endoscopic "rigid" plastic stents are used only for pancreatic and biliary indications use, while expandable metal stents are used in the biliary tree (rarely in the pancreas) and the remaining areas in the gastrointestinal tract. With technological advances in guidewires, stent and endoscope design stents are now used for the palliation and definitive treatment of benign and malignant disease of the pancreaticobiliary and gastrointestinal tract.

Gastrointest Endoscopy Clin N Am 21 (2011) xv–xvi
doi:10.1016/j.giec.2011.04.013
1052-5157/11/$ – see front matter

I have been fortunate to witness the evolution of gastrointestinal stents. As a first-year endoscopy fellow in 1991, I recall being involved in the placement of a rigid esophageal stent for palliation of malignant dysphagia and as a third-tier biliary fellow in 1993 being involved with the placement of an expandable metal biliary stent, which had only recently become FDA approved for endoscopic palliation. Shortly after completion of my fellowship, FDA-approved expandable esophageal stents became available. We subsequently used esophageal and biliary stents for gastric, duodenal, and colonic use as the development of stents specifically for these latter indications did not come for several more years. It has been satisfying to be able to use plastic and metal stents to positively impact the clinical course of ill patients and in many cases have achieved dramatic clinical improvements after placing them for palliative, preoperative, and curative intents.

In this issue of *Gastrointestinal Endoscopy Clinics of North America* a series of articles are published that review the use of rigid and expandable metal stents throughout the gastrointestinal tract. As an overview, the initial article discusses tissue responses to expandable stents. Separate articles on the use of expandable stents for benign esophageal and biliary disease, malignant esophageal and biliary disease, and malignant colonic obstruction are included. Likewise, separate articles on rigid plastic stent use for benign and malignant biliary indications and for pancreatic use are discussed. Finally, the use of expandable stents in unusual locations is presented.

It is hoped that the information in this issue will increase your understanding of stent use that will translate into improvement in patient care. Along the way it is also hoped that you will be able to appreciate the historical aspects of stent development.

Todd H. Baron, MD
Division of Gastroenterology and Hepatology
Department of Medicine
Mayo Clinic
Rochester, MN 55905, USA

E-mail address:
baron.todd@mayo.edu

REFERENCES

1. Sterioff S. Etymology of the world "stent". Mayo Clin Proc 1997;72(4):377–9.
2. Esser JF. Studies in plastic surgery of the face: I. Use of skin from the neck to replace face defects. II. Plastic operations about the mouth. III. The epidermic inlay. Ann Surg 1917;65(3):297–315.
3. Re Mine WH, Grindlay JH. Skinlined omentum and plastic sponge tubes for experimental choledochoduodenostomy. AMA Arch Surg 1954;69(2):255–62.
4. Molnar W, Stockum AE. Relief of obstructive jaundice through percutaneous trans-hepatic catheter—a new therapeutic method. Am J Roentgenol Radium Ther Nucl Med 1974;122(2):356–67.
5. Soehendra N, Reynders-Frederix V. Palliative biliary duct drainage. A new method for endoscopic introduction of a new drain. Dtsch Med Wochenschr 1979;104(6): 206–7 [in German].

Expandable Metal Stents: Principles and Tissue Responses

Nimish Vakil, MD[a,b,*]

KEYWORDS

• Metal stents • Expandable stents • Biodegradable stents
• Removable stents

Expandable metal stents revolutionized the treatment of malignant stenoses in the gastrointestinal tract. These devices were originally designed for intravascular application, and the earliest studies used vascular stents to demonstrate feasibility of use in the gastrointestinal tract. In the biliary tree, these devices allowed placement of stents that open to a much wider diameter than conventional plastic stents, and the flexible delivery systems and the pliability of the stent materials allowed them to be placed in areas where rigid plastic stents were more difficult to use. In the esophagus, placement of rigid plastic stents often required general anesthesia and was associated with high complication and mortality rates. Expandable stents allow outpatient placement with low complication rates.[1] The flexibility of these stents and the precise positioning allow them to be placed at locations that were traditionally difficult to stent, such as stenoses close to the upper esophageal sphincter.[2] These devices also opened the era of stenting in nontraditional areas, such as the colon and the duodenum, where rigid stents cannot be used. An understanding of the tissue responses to metal stents led to the development of partially covered stents that would resist tumor ingrowth into the stent lumen and development of fully covered stents that could be removed after a period of time because they do not integrate into the wall of the organ. Finally, biodegradable stents are now available that react with tissue in a different way and disintegrate after a period of time. Each of the stent designs has specific applications, risks, and benefits that must be matched to the needs of patients.

PRINCIPLES OF EXPANDABLE STENT PLACEMENT

The general principle of all expandable stents is to provide a wide lumen without the complications of passing a large introducer system through a stenosis. This prevents

[a] University of Wisconsin School of Medicine and Public Health, Madison WI, USA
[b] Department of Gastroenterology, Aurora Summit Hospital, WI, USA
* Aurora Summit Hospital, 36500 Aurora Drive, Summit, WI 53066.
E-mail address: nvakil@wisc.edu

Gastrointest Endoscopy Clin N Am 21 (2011) 351–357
doi:10.1016/j.giec.2011.04.008
1052-5157/11/$ – see front matter © 2011 Elsevier Inc. All rights reserved.

giendo.theclinics.com

complications, such as perforation. Therefore, expandable stents are either provided preloaded on a delivery system with the stent constrained or must be constrained onto a delivery system before being deployed. Stents are most often placed by a combination of endoscopy and fluoroscopy, but in some tumor locations and clinical situations, stents may be placed by fluoroscopy or endoscopy alone.

Stricture Dilation Before Stent Placement

Stricture dilation is occasionally necessary in cases of extremely tight stenosis but it is important to avoid overdilating the stenosis because this can increase the risk of stent migration.

Selecting a Stent of Sufficient Length

In a malignant stenosis, the stent should be long enough to straddle the tumor and long enough to prevent the possibility of tumor overgrowth along the length of the stent. In special locations, precise stent lengths are critical for success. At the gastroesophageal junction, excessive stent length in the body of the stomach increases the risk of migration and impaction against the greater curvature as peristalsis works on the trailing edge of the stent.

Radial Force of the Stent

Stents vary in the degree of radial force exerted. This may be relevant in some circumstances. In patients undergoing chemoradiation for esophageal cancer, stents with high radial force can cause necrosis of the wall of the esophagus and result in serious complications.[3] With high cervical strictures, stents with high radial force can cause stridor due to tracheal compression if a stent has not been previously placed in the trachea.[2]

Stent Shape and Architecture

Flaring the proximal and distal ends of a stent decreases the risk of migration but some stent designs have had widely flared proximal ends that increase tissue hyperplasia. Sharp wires at the ends of the stent can cause tissue reactions by embedding themselves into the mucosa and have generally been replaced by smoother profiles at the ends of the stent.

Uncovered, Covered, and Partially Covered Stents

The choice of stent design depends on the location of the stent, the anticipated life expectancy of the patient, potential treatments, and the biology of the tumor. Only general principles can be offered due to the many variables involved in decision making. In malignant stenoses, tumor ingrowth needs to be balanced against the risk of migration caused by treatment-induced necrosis of the tumor. Tissue responses to the stent are discussed later and additional details are provided about the principles of stent selection.

TISSUE RESPONSES TO STENTS
Animal Studies of Stent Placement

Animal studies have shown variable tissue responses. These studies provided the initial insight that the stent wires can deeply imbed and move from the lumen into the wall of the organ and beyond. In dogs, an uncovered Wallstent (5-mm diameter) was shown to result in extensive fibrosis in the wall of the bile duct.[4] There was marked hyperplasia of the normal mucosa at the proximal and distal ends of the stent. The stent migrated deep into the muscularis and was close to the serosal surface. In the pig, an 18-mm nitinol stent caused necrosis of the mucosa and submucosa with the stent eroding into the muscular layer of the esophagus.[5]

Human Tissue Responses to Stent Placement

Human tissue responses are difficult to study because tissue samples are hard to obtain after stent placement. Furthermore, histologic examination of the tissues with an implanted stent requires special microtomes that can cut through metal without damaging the delicate tissues that surround the stent. Limited data are, therefore, available from human tissue responses to expandable stents.[6,7]

TIME COURSE OF EVENTS AFTER PLACEMENT OF EXPANDABLE STENTS
Metal Stents

Metal stents are available as uncovered, partially covered, or fully covered stents. An uncovered stent consists of a mesh that is bare and expands into the stenosis. A completely covered stent consists of a mesh stent that is covered by a membrane throughout its length. A partially covered stent consists of a stent with a membrane covering and uncovered proximal and distal ends of the stent.

Uncovered metal stents
Based on our studies in which organs with indwelling stents were removed at surgery or autopsy and examined histologically, differing sequences of events with the uncovered, covered, and partially covered stents are proposed.[6,7]

Initial changes
When an uncovered metal stent expands, the wire of the stent expands into the malignant tumor and abuts against the normal mucosa at the proximal and distal ends of the stent.[6,7] The radial force of the stent causes necrosis of superficial layers of the tumor and the superficial layers of the mucosa as the stent erodes into the submucosa of the organ (**Fig. 1**). An inflammatory exudate covers the luminal aspect of the stent and a few inflammatory cells are seen around the struts of the stent. In the tumor mass, the stent erodes into the tumor and tumor tissue overhangs the struts of the stent (see **Fig. 1**). Fully covered stents exert radial pressure on the tumor and on the normal mucosa above and below the tumor.[6,7] The pressure exerted by the stent causes ischemic necrosis of the tumor and the normal mucosa. A fibrinous exudate develops in response and some fibrosis occurs at the surface of the normal mucosa but the membrane bonded to the stent material prevents imbedding of the stent into the submucosa (**Fig. 2**). This status quo is preserved as long as the membrane remains bonded to the material of the stent. If the membrane separates from the stent material, the resultant uncovered areas can migrate into the submucosa and eventually become integrated into the organ making removal of the stent difficult. Fully covered stents can be placed in benign stenoses. Their radial force dilates the stricture and the fully covered design prevents the stent from becoming integrated into the wall of the organ and allowing removability.[6,7] Partially covered stents (**Fig. 3**) have properties of both covered and uncovered stent types. The uncovered portions of the stent at the proximal and distal ends behave like any other uncovered stent. The midportion of the stent is membrane covered and straddles the tumor preventing ingrowth of tumor tissue.

Late changes after stent placement
One month after stent placement, fibrosis develops in response to pressure necrosis caused by the radial force of the stent.[6,7] With an uncovered stent, the fibrosis can cover the sent integrating it into the wall of the organ. The entire stent may no longer be visible after several months of placement. In the tumor mass itself, tumor tissue

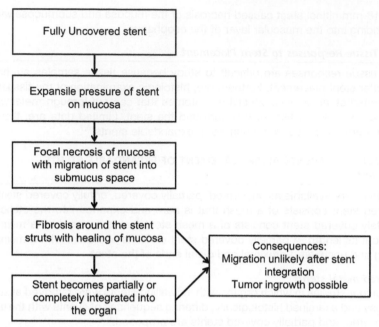

Fig. 1. Tissue responses to uncovered expandable stents and subsequent consequences.

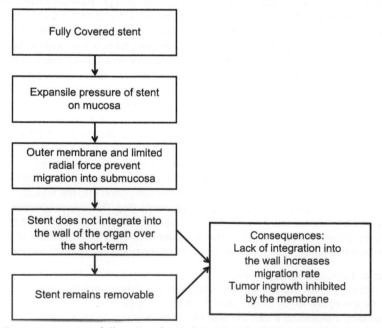

Fig. 2. Tissue responses to fully covered metal stents and subsequent consequences.

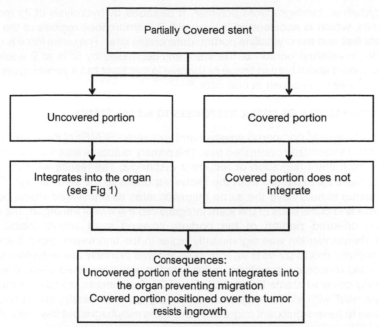

Fig. 3. Tissue responses to partially covered stents and subsequent consequences.

overgrows the struts of the stent in untreated patients. In patients who receive chemoradiation, fibrosis replaces tumor tissue and the stent becomes enmeshed in the fibrous tissue.

Tissue overgrowth at the ends of the stent
Stents are often flared at their proximal and distal ends. Due to the higher radial pressure at these sites, the tissue reaction is exaggerated and an exuberant amount of fibrous material can cause stent occlusion. Some stent designs predispose to the development of granulation tissue. Pointed stent wires that are exposed and turned outwards can drive into the mucosa and cause a greater tissue reaction.

Special Circumstances

Stents before and after chemoradiation
Chemotherapy can cause necrosis of the tumor and radiation can cause injury to the normal mucosa above and below the stent. Radiation causes extensive sloughing and ulceration of the mucosa and the muscular wall of the esophagus can become markedly thinner and replaced by fibrous tissue. Stents with high radial pressure can cause extensive necrosis and in organs, such as the esophagus, the scarred wall, which can be quite thin, may necrose completely, resulting in the stent eroding into the mediastinum. Fatal hemorrhage from stent erosion into the aorta has been reported as has a paraspinal abscess.

BIODEGRADABLE STENTS

The Ella stent (ELLA-CS, Hradec Králové, Czech Republic) is a biodegradable stent that is approved for use in Europe and some parts of Asia.[8] It is made from commercially available polydioxanone absorbable surgical suture material. Polydioxanone is a semicrystalline, biodegradable polymer. It degrades by hydrolysis of its molecule ester bonds, which is accelerated by low pH. The amorphous regions of the matrix deteriorate first and the crystalline portion deteriorates later. The radial force is dependent on the crystalline portion of the stent and decreases by 50% at 9 weeks. Not enough is known about human tissue responses to this stent but a severe hyperplastic reaction has been described in one case.[8]

CLINICAL CORRELATES OF TISSUE RESPONSES TO METAL STENTS

Vakil and colleagues[9] compared covered and uncovered SEMSs of identical design in a multicenter randomized controlled trial. The primary outcome was the need for reintervention from stent migration or recurrent dysphagia. The results were consistent with what might be expected from the tissue responses to the stent design. Partially covered stents should have the same migration rates as uncovered stents because the proximal and distal ends of the stent integrate into the wall of the organ. The central membrane covered portion of the partially covered stent should inhibit tumor ingrowth. Reintervention was significantly higher in the uncovered group than in the partially covered group (27 vs 0 %, $P = .002$) and was primarily due to tumor ingrowth or obstructing mucosal hyperplasia, more common with uncovered stents compared with partially covered stents (30 vs 3 %, $P = .005$). Both stents provided comparable dysphagia relief with similar migration rates. Fully covered plastic stents have also been shown to have significant migration rates in the esophagus but low rates of tumor ingrowth.[10,11]

In distal bile duct obstruction, partially covered metal stents have been compared with uncovered stents.[12,13] Migration rates are higher with covered stents and tumor ingrowth is greater with uncovered stents.

In summary, tissue responses to stents predict clinical responses to metal stents. Further studies are required on tissue responses to biodegradable stents and covered removable plastic stents.

REFERENCES

1. Knyrim K, Wagner HJ, Bethge N, et al. A controlled trial of an expansile metal stent for palliation of esophageal obstruction due to inoperable cancer. N Engl J Med 1993;329(18):1302–7.
2. Bethge N, Sommer A, Vakil N. A prospective trial of self-expanding metal stents in the palliation of malignant esophageal strictures near the upper esophageal sphincter. Gastrointest Endosc 1997;45(3):300–3.
3. Bethge N, Sommer A, von Kleist D, et al. A prospective trial of self-expanding metal stents in the palliation of malignant esophageal obstruction after failure of primary curative therapy. Gastrointest Endosc 1996;44(3):283–6.
4. Silvis SE, Sievert CE Jr, Vennes JA, et al. Comparison of covered versus uncovered wire mesh stents in the canine biliary tract. Gastrointest Endosc 1994;40(1): 17–21.
5. Cwikiel W, Willén R, Stridbeck H, et al. Self-expanding stent in the treatment of benign esophageal strictures: experimental study in pigs and presentation of clinical cases. Radiology 1993;187(3):667–71.
6. Bethge N, Sommer A, Gross U, et al. Human tissue responses to metal stents implanted in vivo for the palliation of malignant stenoses. Gastrointest Endosc 1996; 43(6):596–602.
7. Vakil N, Gross U, Bethge N. Human tissue responses to metal stents. Gastrointest Endosc Clin N Am 1999;9(3):359–65.

8. Hair CS, Devonshire DA. Severe hyperplastic tissue stenosis of a novel biode-gradable esophageal stent and subsequent successful management with high-pressure balloon dilation. Endoscopy 2010;42(Suppl 2):E132–3.
9. Vakil N, Morris AI, Marcon N, et al. A prospective, randomized, controlled trial of covered expandable metal stents in the palliation of malignant esophageal obstruction at the gastroesophageal junction. Am J Gastroenterol 2001;96(6): 1791–6.
10. Bethge N, Vakil N. A prospective trial of a new self-expanding plastic stent for malignant esophageal obstruction. Am J Gastroenterol 2001;96(5):1350–4.
11. Repici A, Vleggaar FP, Hassan C, et al. Efficacy and safety of biodegradable stents for refractory benign esophageal strictures: the BEST (Biodegradable Esophageal Stent) study. Gastrointest Endosc 2010;72(5):927–34.
12. Kullman E, Frozanpor F, Söderlund C, et al. Covered versus uncovered self-expandable nitinol stents in the palliative treatment of malignant distal biliary obstruction: results from a randomized, multicenter study. Gastrointest Endosc 2010;72(5):915–23.
13. Telford JJ, Carr-Locke DL, Baron TH, et al. A randomized trial comparing uncov-ered and partially covered self-expandable metal stents in the palliation of distal malignant biliary obstruction. Gastrointest Endosc 2010;72(5):907–14.

Expandable Stents for Benign Esophageal Disease

Kulwinder S. Dua, MD, FRCP (Edinburgh), FRCP (London)

KEYWORDS
- Self-expandable esophageal metal stent
- Self-expandable esophageal plastic stent
- Biodegradable stent • Refractory benign esophageal stricture
- Esophageal perforation • Esophageal leak • Esophageal fistula
- Achalasia

The efficacy of self-expanding metal stents (SEMSs) in the palliation of malignant esophageal diseases has been extensively studied and published. With a greater than 95% technical success rate in placement and almost immediate relief in symptoms, SEMSs have become the most widely accepted modality used to palliate malignant dysphagia and/or malignant esophageal fistulae.[1–8] Compared with the previous semirigid plastic tubes, which were associated with higher complication rates,[4,5,8,9] SEMSs have a smaller diameter delivery catheter; thus, preinsertion dilatation of the esophageal stricture is not required in most patients. Despite this smaller diameter, once released, these stents can expand to large diameters; the expansion is gradual rather than abrupt and the stent can conform to the shape of the stricture. Where required, it is easy to deploy another stent into a previously placed stent. To prevent tumor in-growth, majority of the SEMS are partially covered with a plastic membrane. Since plastic covering makes SEMS susceptible to migration, the uncovered segments at the upper and lower ends of the stent allow for tissue in-growth and embedment (**Fig. 1**). Although this makes the stent nonremovable, removability is a not an issue when stents are used in patients with limited life expectancy. Experience in using SEMSs in those with limited life expectancy has also not given opportunity to evaluate their efficacy when used on a long-term basis. A study from the MD Anderson Cancer Center in Houston, Texas, showed that if SEMSs are kept in place for several weeks, even for malignant indications, patients can start experiencing significant and life-threatening complication (37%); a suggestion has been made that palliation of malignant dysphagia may be better accomplished by a combination

Conflict of interest statement: The author is the inventor of the antireflux valve for which he has a patent assignment agreement with Cook Endoscopy.
Division of Gastroenterology and Hepatology, Department of Medicine, Medical College of Wisconsin, 9200 West Wisconsin Avenue, Milwaukee, WI 53226, USA
E-mail address: kdua@mcw.edu

Gastrointest Endoscopy Clin N Am 21 (2011) 359–376
doi:10.1016/j.giec.2011.04.001
1052-5157/11/$ – see front matter © 2011 Elsevier Inc. All rights reserved.

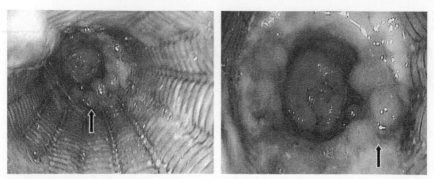

Fig. 1. Tissue in-growth into the lower uncovered segment of a partially covered self-expanding metal esophageal stent (*arrows*) (Ultraflex stent, Boston Scientific, Natick, MA).

of SEMS (immediate symptom relief) with brachytherapy and removal of SEMS after 4 to 6 weeks to avoid complications.[10,11]

With uncertainties regarding removability and complications associated with long-term use, SEMSs have not received widespread acceptance for benign esophageal disorders. Initial experience has been discouraging primarily because of granulation tissue in-growth into the uncovered part of SEMSs (see **Fig. 1**) as well as tissue embedment, making them difficult, if not impossible, to remove. Newer SEMSs that are fully covered, hence do not embed, are now available. These stents seem removable but are still not approved for benign indications. Recently, a fully covered self-expanding plastic esophageal stent (SEPS) (Polyflex, Boston Scientific, Natick, MA, USA) made of woven plastic strands (potentially inducing less tissue reaction compared with metal) was developed. This stent can be removed and is Food and Drug Administration (FDA) approved for treatment of benign refractory esophageal strictures. Another attractive concept has been the introduction of biodegradable stents, where the issue of removability does not exist because these stents eventually undergo metabolic degradation and absorption. With the availability of SEPSs, fully covered SEMSs (FC-SEMSs), and biodegradable stents, interest in using expandable stents for benign esophageal disorders has been revived. This review focuses on experience in using self-expanding stents for benign esophageal diseases with special emphasis on refractory benign esophageal strictures (RBESs) and benign esophageal perforations, leaks, and fistulae.

REFRACTORY BENIGN ESOPHAGEAL STRICTURES

Before embarking on endotherapy for esophageal stricture, it is important to establish that the stricture is benign by multiple biopsies and by imaging studies where needed. Similarly, it is important to address the primary cause of the stricture. For example, a peptic stricture is labeled as refractory if a patient is not receiving or is not compliant with strict antireflux measures. In addition to cause, the stricture anatomic characteristics may have influence on the outcomes of endotherapy. Benign esophageal strictures can either be classified as simple (short [<2 cm], straight, and wide enough to allow a standard 9.5-mm diameter endoscope to pass) or complex (long [>2 m], tortuous, multiple sites, and too narrow to allow passage of a standard endoscope). Besides esophageal rings and webs, simple strictures are generally peptic in origin whereas complex strictures can develop after corrosive injuries, radiation therapy, surgery, and esophageal ablative treatments, such as photodynamic therapy and mucosal resections.

Endoscopic dilatation using a bougie or balloon dilators is the most widely accepted method for treating benign esophageal strictures. Up to 40% of benign strictures may recur,[12] requiring periodic dilatations. Simple strictures tend to respond better to dilatations and eventually the intervals between periodic dilatations become longer. Complex strictures, alternatively, are difficult to treat, carry a higher procedural complication rate, and tend to recur within weeks.[13,14] These strictures are considered RBESs. Various investigators have defined RBESs in different ways and this may have had some bearing on the confounding results of endotherapy published in the literature. To standardize the characteristics of RBESs, Kochman and colleagues[15] proposed the following definition: an anatomic fibrotic esophageal restriction, absence of inflammation or motility disorder, and inability to achieve a diameter of greater than or equal to 14 mm in 5 sessions of dilatations at 2-week intervals or inability to maintain a diameter of greater than or equal to 14 mm for 4 weeks once greater than or equal 14-mm diameter is achieved. This definition does not address the influence of the cause of the strictures on the outcomes of therapy because RBES from corrosive injury may behave differently from RBES secondary to radiation therapy.

Besides repeated high-risk dilatations, several endoscopic approaches have been tried for treating RBES. Some of these include intralesional steroid injection, electrocautery incision, argon-plasma coagulation, expandable stents, and a combination of these modalities. Surgeries with associated morbidity and mortality or gastrostomy tube feeding are alternatives for those not responding to endoscopic interventions.

The Concept of Using Expandable Stents for RBESs

If during endoscopic dilatation, a few seconds of stretching with a bougie or a balloon can relieve dysphagia for a few weeks, then, conceptually speaking, stretching the stricture continuously with a dilator in place for several weeks may give longer-lasting benefit by allowing tissue to remold around the dilator. Expandable esophageal stents are ideal in achieving this because they not only function as dilators but also maintain luminal patency while stretching the stricture continuously for weeks (**Fig. 2**). Unlike for malignant strictures, one of the major issues for using stents for benign indications is the need to subsequently remove the stent. The types of self-expanding esophageal stents that have been used for RBESs are metal stents (partially covered and fully covered), plastic stents, and biodegradable stents. Unfortunately, most of the studies evaluating these stents for RBESs have been small, retrospective case series and there have been no major prospective, randomized studies comparing various alternative endoscopic techniques with stenting or comparing one type of stent with another type. Similarly, no major conclusions can be made on the influence of the cause of RBESs on the outcomes from stenting because most of the case series are small and included patients with RBESs from a variety of causes.

Partially Covered Self-Expanding Esophageal Metal Stent

Partially covered SEMSs (PC-SEMSs) have been primarily designed for malignant esophageal strictures. Although they can be uncovered, the majority of SEMSs used are those coated with plastic to prevent tumor in-growth. To reduce the risks of migration, short segments at the upper and lower ends of the stent are left uncovered for tissue in-growth and tissue embedment to allow for better anchoring (see **Fig. 1**). Tissue embedding of SEMSs was demonstrated by Bethge and colleagues[16] and, although this feature reduces the risks of migration, it makes removal of

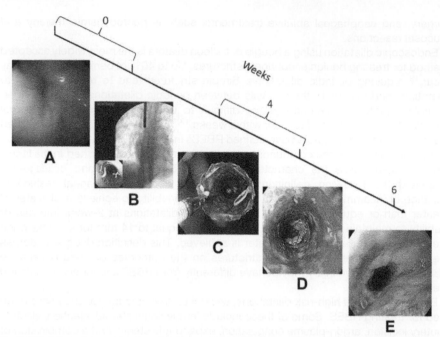

Fig. 2. (*A*) A 3 cm long refractory benign esophageal stricture in a 4-year old child secondary to corrosive ingestion. (*B*) A 12 mm diameter and 70 mm long fully covered self-expanding metal esophageal stent was deployed across the stricture (Alimaxx-ES stent, Merit Medicals, UT, USA). This 12 mm diameter fully covered stent was recently released for use in malignant strictures and is not FDA cleared for benign esophageal strictures. It was used in this child because the minimum 16 mm diameter Polyflex stent (only stent FDA cleared for use in benign stricture in the US; Boston Scientific, Natick, MA) would have been too large for this child. (*C*) Four weeks after placement the stent was easily removed and, (*D*) on endoscopy the previously narrowed segment appeared adequately dilated and showed mucosal ulceration. (*E*) Repeat endoscopy 2 weeks later showed significant healing of the mucosal ulceration.

PC-SEMSs difficult and a high-risk procedure. This may not be an issue when PC-SEMSs are placed permanently for palliation of malignant dysphagia. For RBESs, if stents are not removed, long-term stent-related complications, including ulceration, bleeding, fistula, and recurrent dysphagia due to migration, granulation tissue, and new stricture formation may occur. Stents may erode into mediastinal structures, including the aorta, with fatal outcomes. PC-SEMSs are not FDA approved for treatment of benign strictures. Nevertheless, anecdotally, PC-SEMSs have been placed in patients with RBESs and there are several small retrospective series in the literature where these stents were associated with poor results. In one series, 4 of 8 patients developed major complications and 1 patient died from bleeding secondary to the stent eroding into the aorta.[17] Similar discouraging results have been reported in several other small series.[18–20] In a review of 29 patients where SEMSs were placed for RBESs, Sandha and colleagues[21] reported an overall complication rate of 80%, which included new stricture formation (40%), migration (31%), and tracheaesophageal fistula (6%).

Due to unacceptable complications associated with tissue in-growth and embedding of the stent, PC SEMSs are not recommended for RBESs.

Fully Covered Self-Expanding Esophageal Metal Stent

Because granulation tissue in-growth into the uncovered segments of PC-SEMSs results in embedment of the stent, one way to overcome this problem is to completely cover the SEMS. Some of the FC-SEMSs available in the United States are listed in **Table 1**. Most of these stents are dog-bone in shape and have a purse-string suture attached at the upper end for repositioning after deployment. This suture or the upper end of the stent can be grasped with a forceps and the stent can be withdrawn using a standard endoscope. Anecdotal and personal experience has shown that these stents can be removed (see **Fig. 2**); as of this review's writing, these stents are not FDA approved for removability. Compared with plastic mesh, the wire mesh design of these stents can be constrained to a thinner diameter; hence, the delivery system of these stents are thinner than a self-expanding plastic stent (SEPS) (Polyflex—the only stent approved by FDA for use in benign strictures). Moreover, unlike the SEPS, these stents are user-friendly because they come preloaded and can be reconstrained during deployment for proper positioning.

In a study on 8 pigs, Baron and colleagues[22] showed that a PC-SEMS (Ultraflex, Boston Scientific) induced severe granulation tissue response embedding the uncovered segments of the stent, making its removal traumatic compared with an FC-SEMS (Alimaxx-ES, Merit Medical, South Jordan, UT, USA) that caused minimal tissue response and could be removed easily without significant trauma. There was, however, a higher migration rate with the FC-SEMSs. Song and colleagues[23] published their study on a new fully covered nitinol SEMS that they placed in 5 patients with benign esophageal strictures. After 2 months, they were successful in removing the stent in all 5 patients with resolution of stricture. The stricture recurred, however, in 2 patients. The same group evaluated the safety and efficacy of this stent in an additional 25 patients with RBESs.[24] The stent was successfully removed in 23 patients at 1 to 8 weeks after insertion. In 2 patients the stent had migrated (passed rectally in one and regurgitated in another). After removal, one patient developed a fistula that closed spontaneously. At mean 13 months' follow up (range 2–25 months), 12 patients remained asymptomatic and in the remaining 13 patients, the strictures recurred requiring dilatations. In a small series of patients with RBESs, Lakhtakia and colleagues[25] were successful in removing the Alimaxx-ES stent after 6 to 12 weeks in place. In another series, 36 Alimaxx-ES stents were placed in 31 patients, of which 7 were for RBESs. Stent removal was successful in all cases where attempted and the success rate in treating RBESs was 29%.[26] In a recent retrospective review, Bakken and colleagues[27] described their experience using an FC-SEMS (Alimaxx-ES) for benign esophageal diseases. There were 25 patients with strictures who underwent a total of 30 procedures. The stent were removed after an average of 67 days (range 0–279 days). Initial success rate in treating strictures was 56%. Stent migration was a major issue that was influenced by the cause of the stricture (radiation 25%, nonradiation 50%, and surgical anastomotic 60%) and the site of stricture (proximal 46%, middle 21%, and distal 38%). Other complications included nausea and emesis requiring hospital visits, neck and chest pain, gastroesophageal reflux, and dysphagia. Life-threatening major complications included stridor during 3 procedures in 2 patients requiring stent removal, respiratory distress in 1 patient (stent removed), and bradycardia/asystole in 1 patient (ICU admission). Another recent smaller retrospective study using Alimaxx-ES stent showed good success rates in treating RBES and fistula with migration rate of 39%.[28]

Based on small case series and retrospective reviews, FC-SEMSs induce minimal tissue reaction and are potentially removable. Initial experience on using these stents

Table 1
Some of the fully covered self-expanding esophageal stents available in the United States

Diameter (mm)	Length (mm)	Delivery Catheter (mm)	Shortening	Recapture	Fully Covered	Company
Self-Expanding Plastic Esophageal Stent (Polyflex Stent)[a]						
16	90, 120, 150	12	Yes	No	Yes	Boston Scientific
18	90, 120, 150	13	Yes	No	Yes	
21	90, 120, 150	14	Yes	No	Yes	
Fully Covered Self-Expanding Metal Esophageal Stent[b]						
Wallflex Stent						
18	103, 123, 153	6.2	Yes	Yes	Yes	Boston Scientific
23	105, 125, 155	6.3	Yes	Yes	Yes	
Alimaxx-ES Stent[c]						
18	70, 100, 120	7.4	No	No	Yes	Merit Medical
22	70, 100, 120	7.4	No	No	Yes	
Evolution Stent						
18	80, 100, 120	8	Yes	Yes	Yes	Cook Endoscopy
20	80, 100, 120	8	Yes	Yes	Yes	
Niti-S Stent[d]						
15	60, 80, 100, 120, 150	5.8	Yes	Yes	Yes	Taewoong Medical
18	60, 80, 100, 120, 150	6.5	Yes	Yes	Yes	
20	60, 80, 100, 120, 150	6.5	Yes	Yes	Yes	

[a] FDA cleared for use in benign esophageal strictures.
[b] Not yet FDA cleared for use in benign esophageal disorders.
[c] Recently, a 12-mm diameter Alimaxx-ES stent was also released by Merit Medicals (see **Fig. 2**).
[d] A 3.5-mm diameter delivery system, through-the scope, fully covered Niti-S esophageal stent is also available.

for RBESs has been encouraging. Influence of the cause on the outcome and the duration for which the stent should be kept in place before removal has not yet been established. Migration has been a major issue and further design modifications are needed. FC-SEMSs are still not FDA cleared for benign indications.

Self-Expanding Esophageal Plastic Stents

The Polyflex stent is an SEPS that can be removed and is FDA approved for treating benign esophageal strictures. The stent is made of polyester mesh with an inner coating of a smooth silicone membrane along the entire length of the stent. Because of the full coating and presumably less tissue reaction to plastic compared with metal, this stent induces minimal granulation tissue formation facilitating easy removal. The upper and lower ends are smoothed by the silicone membrane to decrease tissue reaction above and below the stent. The proximal end is flared out to reduce the chances of migration. Since the stent is made of plastic, to enhance radiological visualization, the plastic is impregnated with barium. Also, there are radiopaque markers located at the upper and lower ends of the stents and an additional marker at the mid-point of the stent. The markers are colored blue for endoscopic positioning. Like SEMSs, SEPSs are available in various diameters and lengths (see **Table 1**). Unlike SEMSs, SEPSs are not preloaded. Using several simple steps, SEPSs are loaded into the delivery catheter and, although this feature may not be as user friendly as SEMSs, it has the advantage of removing, reloading, and reusing the same stent if deployed incorrectly. Unfortunately, the diameter of the delivery system is large (12 mm, 13 mm, and 14 mm for 16-mm, 18-mm, and 21-mm diameter stents, respectively), hence preinsertion dilatation is required in almost all patients. A newer SEPS is being developed to overcome some of these limitations. Unlike SEMSs, there is no suture at the upper end and the stent is removed by grabbing a spot on the upper rim of the stent and slowly withdrawing it.

Repici and colleagues[29] treated 15 patients with esophageal strictures who had failed prior repeated dilatations. SEPSs could be placed in all patients and removed from all patients after 6 weeks. At a mean follow-up of 22.7 months, 12 patients (80%) remained symptom-free. There was one stent migration. In a slightly larger retrospective review, Evrard and colleagues[30] found SEPSs curative in 17 of 21 patients with RBES at mean 21 (range 8–39) months' follow-up. The stent could be removed in all patients and there was one major complication of tracheal compression requiring stent removal.

Subsequent experience from other centers using SEPSs for RBESs could not reproduce the results (discussed previously).[31–35] On the contrary, studies showed poor cure rates with significant associated complication rates, which included migration, hemorrhage, chest pain, ulceration, and esophageal perforation. In a small series of 5 patients treated with SEPSs, all developed complications in the form of migration, chest pain, and one perforation.[32] In another retrospective review, Holm reported a low success rate of only 6%.[31] Complications included chest pain, nausea/emesis, and dysphagia. Stent migration was noted in up to 82% and was more common with proximal and distal stent placements compared with the midesophagus.

The exact reason for the excellent results from Europe and poor results from other centers is not clear. These variable results could be due to the studies enrolling patients with different definitions of RBES, different case mixes, variable periods for which the stents were kept in place and the retrospective nature of the design. To address some of these issues, a prospective (nonrandomized) study was conducted in which 40 patients were enrolled.[36] All these patients fulfilled the definition of RBES.[15] A SEPS (Polyflex) was deployed across the stricture and then removed after

4 to 6 weeks. Technical success rates of stent placement and removal were 93% and 94%, respectively. At a median of 53 weeks (range 11–153) follow-up, 30% (intention to treat) of patients were dysphagia-free. Another 30% of patients with recurrence of dysphagia after stent removal opted for insertion of a new Polyflex stent for a longer duration rather than returning to their baseline alternatives of repeated frequent dilations, gastrostomy tube feeding, or surgery. This approach was able to change the outcomes from baseline alternatives in 66% of patients, which also included those who did not want the stent to be removed. Unfortunately, complications in the form of migration (22%), severe chest pain (11%), bleeding (8%), and perforation (5.5%) were observed. One patient who refused stent removal died of severe bleeding probably related to an aortoesophageal fistula. A recent study compared Polyflex stents with repeated dilations. Both approaches were equally effective in relieving dysphagia but the Polyflex stent group required a lower number of dilations.[37] In a pooled-data analysis of 10 studies using SEPSs for RBESs that involved a total of 130 patients, Repici and colleagues[38] found that SEPSs were successfully inserted in 128 of 130 patients (98%). Clinical success using this approach was achieved in 68 patients (52%; 95% CI, 44%–61%) with a lower success rates in those with a cervical strictures (33% success rate in treating cervical strictures vs 54% for other sites; $P<.05$). Major complications occurred in 12 patients (9%; 95% CI, 4%–14%), resulting in one death (0.8%). Other complications included early (<4 weeks) migration in 19 patients (24%; 95% CI, 14%–32%), and 25 patients (21%) required postinsertion endoscopic reinterventions.

With the available data, the optimum duration for which SEPSs should remain in place is not certain. Although cleared by the FDA and approved for use in benign esophageal strictures for duration of up to 270 days, this approach can be associated with significant complication rates and should be considered in select patients and preferably in a protocol setting.

Biodegradable Esophageal Stents

Biodegradable stents are made of material that can be metabolized (polylactide/poly-dioxanone) by the body; hence, these stents do not need manual removal. The stents are uncovered, and tissue in-growth, if it occurs, can anchor the stent. Currently, Ella-CS, in Králové, Czech Republic, manufactures biodegradable stents of various lengths and diameters (**Table 2**). Stents are packaged separately and require manual loading immediately before insertion. The stents are flexible and have radiopaque markers at the ends. There are limited data on their loss of radial force over time. According to company specifications, the stents maintain integrity and radial force for 6 to 8 weeks after placement and disintegration occurs by 11 to 12 weeks. Low pH (as can occur with gastroesophageal reflux) accelerates disintegration.

Table 2
Biodegradable esophageal stent (SX-ELLA biodegradable stent)

Diameter (mm)	Length (mm)	Delivery Catheter (mm)	Preloaded	Fully Covered	Company
16	60, 80, 100	Proximal 5.9	No (stent is	No	Ella-CS
18	60, 80, 100	Distal 9.4	manually loaded	No	(Králové,
23	60, 80, 100		immediately	No	Czech
25	60, 80, 100, 135		before placement)	No	Republic)

Saito and colleagues[39] made a biodegradable stent by knitting poly-L-lactic acid monofilaments. They placed this stent in 13 patients (corrosive injury in 2, postsurgery in 4, and postendoscopic mucosal dissection in 7). Spontaneous migration occurred in 10 of 13 patients at 10 to 21 days postplacement. At 7 to 24 months' follow-up, all patients were symptom-free. The same group was successful in treating 2 patients with strictures secondary to endoscopic mucosal dissection using biodegradable stents.[40] A polydioxanone biodegradable stent (SX-ELLA BD stent, Ella-CS, Králové, Czech Republic) was placed in 4 patients with RBES.[41] On follow-up endoscopic evaluation, stent disintegration was noted at 10 to 12 weeks after placement. During a short follow-up period of 4 to 17 weeks, all patients were dysphagia-free. In a recent prospective study from 2 European centers, 21 patients with RBES, as defined as Kochman and colleagues,[15] were enrolled.[42] A biodegradable stent (SX-ELLA) was placed and patients were clinically and endoscopically followed-up for 6 months and then only when symptoms recurred. Apart from 2 patients in whom the stent migrated, the stent was found fragmented in all patients endoscopically 3 months after deployment. At a median follow-up of 53 weeks (range 25–88), 45% patients were dysphagia-free. Severe pain (2 patients) and minor bleeding (1 patient) were some of the complications that occurred. Case reports of new esophageal fistula and tissue hyperplasia have been reported with biodegradable stents.[43,44]

NONMALIGNANT ESOPHAGEAL PERFORATIONS, LEAKS, AND FISTULAE

Esophageal perforation can occur during endoscopic procedures, such as dilatation or mucosal resection/dissection. These perforations are usually recognized immediately and appropriate interventions can be applied before mediastinal contamination occurs. These patients may not require mediastinal drainage and their prognosis is better than those in whom mediastinitis develops from delay in diagnosis as can occur with spontaneous perforation (eg, Boerhaave syndrome). Leaks are generally seen at surgical anastomotic sites and these leaks can evolve into fistulae.

Surgery is considered the gold standard in treating patients with esophageal perforations and leaks. Surgery can be associated, however, with significant morbidity and mortality, especially in the elderly with multiple comorbidities.[45–48] As an alternative to surgery, endoscopic options include placement of expandable covered metal stents, clips, suturing, application of tissue glue, or a combination of these options.[49] Some of the advantages of the endoscopic approach are (1) it is minimally invasive; thus hospital stay is potentially shorter; (2) it can be applied immediately after perforation is recognized during or after an endoscopic procedure; (3) it can allow for early oral intake if esophagram shows no leakage; (4) it does not preclude subsequent surgery if needed; and (5) because iatrogenic perforations often occur during dilatation of strictures, endotherapy with stents can also be used to manage the underlying stricture.

Similar to RBES, there are no major prospective randomized studies comparing endotherapy with surgery or even comparing the various endoscopic techniques with each other. In a recent retrospective review of 125 patients with esophageal perforations, those treated with expandable stents had lower mortality compared with those who underwent esophageal resection.[50] Uncovered expandable stents should not be used to seal perforations/leaks or fistulae for obvious reasons. Because PC-SEMSs are associated with prohibitive complication rates (as discussed previously, with RBESs), they should preferably be avoided. In a recent study, all 4 patients who had PC-SEMSs placed for esophageal perforation suffered perforation during attempted stent removal at approximately 29 days after placement.[51] Biodegradable stents are uncovered, hence not ideal for perforations and leaks. SEMSs or SEPSs can offer a minimally invasive alternative to surgery.

Several small case series have evaluated the feasibility and efficacy of expandable esophageal stents in the treatment of esophageal perforations, leaks, and fistulae.[3,35,45,52–61] Using large-diameter covered expandable stents (Flamingo Wallstent [Boston Scientific], 30-mm flange diameter and 20-mm body diameter, and Ultraflex stent, 28-mm and 23-mm flange and body diameters respectively), Siersema and colleagues[57] treated 11 patients with traumatic perforations (Boerhaave syndrome in 5 patients) where the median time between perforation and endotherapy was 60 hours (24 hours to 28 days). Secondary to this delay, a chest drain was placed in all patients. The perforation was sealed in 10 patients. One of these patients required surgery for incomplete drainage of the pleural cavity and the mediastinum. Of the remaining 9 patients, the stent was removed in 7 after a median of 7 weeks (2 refused removal). In another series, perforation closure was successful in 12 of 13 patients with stent removal or replacement performed after 3 weeks.[59] A total of 17 covered SEMSs were removed with no complications. The patient who did not respond died after an open esophageal diversion procedure. In a study specifically examining iatrogenic perforations, 17 patients were enrolled (8 patients postendoscopy perforation and 9 patients postsurgery).[53] Covered expandable stents were used and the leak was successfully closed in 16 (94%) cases with 14 patients resuming oral intake within 72 hours. One patient with continued leakage underwent surgery. Stent migration requiring repositioning or replacement occurred in 3 patients (18%). Median hospital stay was 5 days and all stents were removed at a mean of 52 ± 20 days. In a recent prospective study, 33 patients with esophageal perforations (iatrogenic in 19 patients, Boerhaave in 10 patients, and other causes in 4 patients) were treated with various types of expandable esophageal stents.[58] A total of 50 stents were placed, of which 45 were SEMSs (90%) and 5 were SEPSs (10%). At initial insertion only 3 stents were fully covered and the remaining 30 stents were partially covered. Complete and immediate sealing of the perforation was observed in 32 (97%) patients. One patient with Boerhaave perforation did not seal with a stent and required surgery. Seven patients died (21%), 4 from uncontrollable sepsis and multiorgan failure. Three of the remaining 26 patients required esophagectomy with stent removal. In the remaining 23 patients, the leak closed at a median of 6 weeks after stent insertion. Thirty-three stents were removed from these 23 patients at a median of 5 weeks after insertion (1–84 weeks). Twenty-three stent extractions were performed within 6 weeks of insertion (group I) and 10 extractions over 6 weeks of insertion (group II). All stent extractions performed in group I were successful without complications whereas 6 complications occurred in 5 patients in group II. These included impacted stents, bleeding, and stent fractures. Because the majority of stents used were PC-SEMSs, this study reinforces the point that partially covered stents become embedded especially if left in place for a longer period of time and extraction not only can be difficult but can be associated with complications.

Similar to iatrogenic and traumatic perforations, stents have been used for spontaneous perforations (Boerhaave syndrome) with encouraging results.[57,58,60,62] SEPSs or covered SEMSs have also been used to successfully close postsurgical anastomotic leaks with success rates reported to be over 80%.[63,64] Life-threatening postsurgery cervical esophageal leaks in 2 patients not fit for reoperation were successfully treated with an FC-SEMS (Alimaxx-ES).[65] In a series of 30 patients with anastomotic leaks treated with SEMSs, the leak successfully closed in 27 (90%) patients.[66] The mean healing time was 30 days. Similar to perforations and leaks, covered expandable esophageal stents have also been used to close benign fistulae. Tracheoesophageal fistulae from prolonged endotracheal intubation in 8 critically ill patients were successfully closed in all patients by inserting a covered SEMS (Ultraflex).[67] The long-term benefit of this approach, however, could not be evaluated because several of these patients died from their primary disease. The stents could easily be removed in 3 patients in whom surgical repair of their fistulae was performed. In one prospective study, 8 of 40 patients with RBES also had fistulae.[36] Using a SEPS (Polyflex stent), successful closure of the fistulae was achieved in 5 (63%) patients.

OTHER BENIGN ESOPHAGEAL CONDITIONS
Achalasia

Li and colleagues[68] recently published long-term follow-up results on 120 patients with achalasia treated either with balloon dilatation (up to 32-mm diameter, 30 patients) or covered SEMSs of varying diameters (20 mm, 25 mm, and 30 mm, with 30 patients in each group). The SEMSs were locally made (Youyan Yijin Advanced Materials, Beijing, People's Republic of China) and remained in place for only 3 to 7 day. All stents were endoscopically removed with a forceps and the investigators used ice-cold water flush to retract the stent before removal. At a mean follow-up of 7 years (range 3–12.7 years) after stent removal, the clinical remission rate in those with the 30-mm SEMS (83.3%) was higher than those in the other groups: balloon dilatation, 0%; 20-mm SEMS, 0%; and 25-mm SEMS, 28.6%. Those treated with the 30-mm SEMS also had greater reduced lower esophageal sphincter pressures compared with the other groups. Despite the stent being in place for short duration, SEMSs migrated in up to 27% of patients with least migration seen in those with a 30-mm SEMS (7%). A significant proportion of patients complained of chest pain (60%–77%) but this was similar to those who underwent balloon dilatation. Other complications in the SEMS group included reflux (up to 23%) and bleeding (up to 17%).

Several recent publications have shown that SEMSs can be successfully used for treating achalasia.[69–71] It seems, however, that the same cohort of patients may have been reported at different times because many of the investigators, including Li and colleagues,[68] are common to all of these publications. It is unclear how 3 to 7 days of stent placement and with significant migration rates can result in several years of clinical remission. In a recent canine study, pneumatic dilatation was associated with significantly more collagen deposition compared with stents.[72] Although an interesting concept, this approach needs further study, especially with commercially available FC-SEMS or SEPS.

Variceal Hemorrhage

Uncontrollable variceal bleeding can be life-threatening, and failure of endoscopic therapy frequently necessitates either placement of a tamponade balloon tube (eg, Sengstaken-Blakemore tube or Minnesota tube) or urgent transjugular intrahepatic portosystemic shun (TIPS). Wright and colleagues[73] recently treated 9 patients with refractory variceal bleeding with SEMSs. Six of the 9 patients survived the acute bleeding episode and the stents were removed endoscopically at a median of 9 days. Stent placement failed to control the bleeding in 3 patients, 2 of whom had gastric varices. In another case report, significant bleeding from a postvariceal banding ulcer was successfully controlled by a covered expandable stent (Ella-ES, Králové, Czech Republic) that was subsequently removed 8 days after placement.[74] Because stents can be placed with endoscopic guidance without fluoroscopy, it is feasible to place SEMSs urgently in an ICU setting. Removal of SEMSs can at times be traumatic, however, and this may have implications in the background of esophageal varices.

SOME TECHNICAL ASPECTS AND CHOOSING A STENT

The same principles that apply to placing expandable stents in malignant strictures apply to RBESs. Patient fitness for the procedure, impending tracheal compression, and stricture characteristics, such as length, location, tightness, and tortuousity, should be determined before the procedure. Because expandable stents can be associated with significant complications and their use for being esophageal indications is not as well established as for malignant conditions, a proper informed consent is essential.

Currently, Polyflex stents (SEPSs) are the only expandable esophageal stents that are FDA approved for use in benign strictures. Polyflex stents require, however, that loading onto the delivery system before the procedure, the delivery system diameter is much larger than pre-loaded FC-SEMSs; thus, preinsertion dilatation of the stricture is required in almost all patients. During deployment, the expanding lower end of the stent tends to eject the remaining stent out of the delivery catheter halfway through deployment. Significant foreshortening and high migration rates are some of the other issues seen with Polyflex stents. SEMSs, alternatively, are preloaded; the delivery catheter has a much smaller diameter, hence an infrequent need for preinsertion dilatation. Some SEMSs (fully covered Wallflex [Boston Scientific, Natick, MA, USA] and Evolution [Cook Endoscopy, Winston Salem, NC, USA]) can be recaptured during deployment for proper positioning, and some do not foreshorten (Alimaxx-ES [Merit Medicals, Salt lake City, UT, USA]) or deploy as proximal release stents (Niti-S [Tae-Woong Medicals, Gomak-RI, Korea]). PC-SEMSs embed into the tissue, thus should not be used as a first-line treatment for benign esophageal disorders. FC-SEMSs are preferable but not yet FDA approved for benign indications.

Because one size or type does not fit all, stent selection should be based on the characters of the stricture, features of the stent, and expertise of the operator. The length of the stent chosen should be long enough to bridge the stricture and have an additional 1.5 cm to 2 cm of stent on either sides of the stricture. Stents with a thinner delivery system are preferable for tight strictures. Compared with a Polyflex stent (delivery catheter diameter 12 mm–14 mm), FC-SEMSs (diameters 5 mm–8 mm) are preferable in these patients. Tight strictures may also require a step-up approach where a thinner diameter stent (eg, 16-mm fully expanded tracheal stent) is first placed and then replaced after a few weeks with larger diameter stents (18 mm or 23 mm). Because some stents can kink when bent,[75] FC-SEMSs (eg, Wallflex and Evolution) that easily conform to the shape of the obstruction are preferable for tortuous strictures. The need for an antireflux mechanism for benign lower esophageal strictures where the stent crosses into the stomach is debatable.[76–79] Strong antireflux measures suffice in most cases. Moreover, the antireflux Z-Stent (Cook Endoscopy; Winston Salem, NC, USA) is partially uncovered and may become embedded. The only antireflux FC-SEMS available is the Niti-S stent. For benign strictures located in the upper esophagus, it is essential to determine the patency of the airways and the possibility of tracheal compression that may require prior airway stenting. Precise positioning of the stent is also essential so as to avoid bridging the upper esophageal sphincter, when not necessary. Possible approaches are the use of nonshortening expandable stents (eg, Alimaxx-ES), proximal release SEMSs (eg, Niti-S stent), and/or close endoscopic monitoring. A partially covered proximal release stent (Ultraflex) is available but with the risk of embedment. Several other stents not yet approved for use in the United States are also available for the proximal esophagus. These stents have a smaller and/or softer upper flange that can also be placed across the upper esophageal sphincter. For situations where the stricture is short (eg, anastomotic ring) or there is minimal to no associated narrowing, as seen in the setting of perforations or leaks, stent migration is a major issue. Some methods used to keep the stent in place are the application of endoscopic clips at the proximal end of the stent to the esophageal wall and, as has been described for malignant strictures, tying a thread to the proximal edge of the stent and then withdrawing the thread through the patient's nostril. To hold the stent in place, the thread is then wrapped around an ear lobule.[80] Generally, larger diameter flange stents should suffice for leaks fistulae and perforations; the larger flange stent also forms a better seal with the esophageal wall minimizing food tracking between the stent and the esophageal wall. At times, even if the stent is not adequately sealing the leak initially, tissue reaction around the stent may eventually close the leak.

Stent removal is generally accomplished endoscopically by grasping the purse-string suture at the upper end of the stent and applying traction. With axial traction, the leading edge and the stretched stent narrow in diameter, facilitating removal. To remove stents that do not have a suture, an edge of the upper end can be grasped with a rat-tooth or longer jaw forceps (pelican or alligator) and removed with traction force using this point as the leading edge. A standard endoscope can be used and it is not essential to use a 2-channel endoscope. Grasping two opposite sites and pulling the stent end-on rather than a leading edge may make negotiating the upper esophageal sphincter difficult.

Partially covered stents have been removed by grasping the lower end of the stent (when free within the stomach) and inverting it on itself. Stents embedded at both the proximal and distal ends are difficult to remove, however. Embedded SEMSs can be removed by thermal (argon plasma coagulation) or mechanical ablation of the in-growing granulation tissue. More recently, removal of embedded PC-SEMS was achieved by placing an FC-SEMS or FC-SPES inside the embedded stent for 7 to 14 days. Pressure necrosis of the tissue between the uncovered portion of the partially covered stent and the covered portion exposes the wires and allows removal of both the stents.[81] In a retrospective review, PC-SEMSs that were placed in 16 patients with RBES were removed using this method. In 91%, both stents were removed in one procedure after a median of 12 days. One procedure was complicated with severe bleeding that was treated endoscopically.

SUMMARY

Partially covered self-expandable esophageal stents are used primarily for palliation of malignant dysphagia and/or fistulae. The feature that helps anchors them in the uncovered segments also renders them nonremovable. Although this may not be an issue in those with limited life expectancy, a nonremovable stent is not an acceptable option for treatment of benign esophageal disorders. Introduction of expandable esophageal stents that can be removed or have the potential for removability has revived interest in using stents for benign esophageal disorders not responding to conventional treatments. The attraction lies in the fact that stents can be placed and removed endoscopically using minimally invasive techniques compared with surgery. Moreover, they do not preclude subsequent surgery in those who do not respond. After deployment, relief of symptoms is immediate but the long-term durability after stent removal is variable. Based on the current literature comprising mostly small retrospective case series, early indications are encouraging for the treatment of

RBESs and esophageal perforations, leaks, and fistulae using SEPSs or FC-SEMSs. The use of partially covered stents is strongly discouraged for treatment of benign indications because tissue in-growth with embedment can result in significant complications. There are few data on the influence of cause of the strictures on outcome of temporary stent placement. There are no comparative studies between the various available stents and the ideal duration for which a stent should be left in place has not been established.

Because expandable esophageal stents can be associated with serious complications when used for benign esophageal disorders, due importance should be given to local expertise and the ability to manage stent-related complications. In addition to considering alternative options, patients should be carefully selected and preferably be enrolled in a protocol.

REFERENCES

1. Bethge N, Knyrim K, Wagner HJ, et al. Self-expanding metal stents for palliation of malignant esophageal obstruction—a pilot study of eight patients. Endoscopy 1992;24(5):411–5.
2. Domschke W, Foerster EC, Matek W, et al. Self-expanding mesh stent for esophageal cancer stenosis. Endoscopy 1990;22:134–6.
3. Fischer A, Thomusch O, Benz S, et al. Nonoperative treatment of 15 benign esophageal perforations with self-expandable covered metal stents. Ann Thorac Surg 2006;81(2):467–72.
4. Gevers AM, Macken E, Hiele M, et al. A comparison of laser therapy, plastic stents, and expandable metal stents for palliation of malignant dysphagia in patients without a fistula. Gastrointest Endosc 1998;48(4):383–8.
5. Knyrim K, Wagner HJ, Bethge N, et al. A controlled trial of an expansile metal stent for palliation of esophageal obstruction due to inoperable cancer. N Engl J Med 1993;329(18):1302–7.
6. Neuhaus H, Hoffmann W, Dittler HJ, et al. Implantation of self-expanding esophageal metal stents for palliation of malignant dysphagia. Endoscopy 1992;24(5):405–10.
7. Ramirez FC, Dennert B, Zierer ST, et al. Esophageal self-expandable metallic stents–indications, practice, techniques, and complications: results of a national survey. Gastrointest Endosc 1997;45(5):360–4.
8. Siersema PD, Hop WC, Dees J, et al. Coated self-expanding metal stents versus latex prostheses for esophagogastric cancer with special reference to prior radiation and chemotherapy: a controlled, prospective study. Gastrointest Endosc 1998;47(2):113–20.
9. Mosca F, Consoli A, Stracqualursi A, et al. Comparative retrospective study on the use of plastic prostheses and self-expanding metal stents in the palliative treatment of malignant strictures of the esophagus and cardia. Dis Esophagus 2003;16(2):119–25.
10. Dua KS. Stents for palliating malignant dysphagia and fistula: is the paradigm shifting? Gastrointest Endosc 2007;65(1):77–81.
11. Ross WA, Alkassab F, Lynch PM, et al. Evolving role of self-expanding metal stents in the treatment of malignant dysphagia and fistulas. Gastrointest Endosc 2007;65(1):70–6.
12. Spechler SJ. American gastroenterological association medical position statement on treatment of patients with dysphagia caused by benign disorders of the distal esophagus. Gastroenterology 1999;117(1):229–33.

13. Said A, Brust DJ, Gaumnitz EA, et al. Predictors of early recurrence of benign esophageal strictures. Am J Gastroenterol 2003;98(6):1252–6.
14. Siersema PD, de Wijkerslooth LR. Dilation of refractory benign esophageal strictures. Gastrointest Endosc 2009;70(5):1000–12.
15. Kochman ML, McClave SA, Boyce HW. The refractory and the recurrent esophageal stricture: a definition. Gastrointest Endosc 2005;62(3):474–5.
16. Bethge N, Sommer A, Gross U, et al. Human tissue responses to metal stents implanted in vivo for the palliation of malignant stenoses. Gastrointest Endosc 1996; 43(6):596–602.
17. Wadhwa RP, Kozarek RA, France RE, et al. Use of self-expandable metallic stents in benign GI diseases. Gastrointest Endosc 2003;58(2):207–12.
18. Ackroyd R, Watson DI, Devitt PG, et al. Expandable metallic stents should not be used in the treatment of benign esophageal strictures. J Gastroenterol Hepatol 2001;16(4):484–7.
19. Fiorini A, Fleischer D, Valero J, et al. Self-expandable metal coil stents in the treatment of benign esophageal strictures refractory to conventional therapy: a case series. Gastrointest Endosc 2000;52(2):259–62.
20. Song HY, Park SI, Do YS, et al. Expandable metallic stent placement in patients with benign esophageal strictures: results of long-term follow-up. Radiology 1997; 203(1):131–6.
21. Sandha GS, Marcon NE. Expandable metal stents for benign esophageal obstruction. Gastrointest Endosc Clin N Am 1999;9(3):437–46.
22. Baron TH, Burgart LJ, Pochron NL. An internally covered (lined) self-expanding metal esophageal stent: tissue response in a porcine model. Gastrointest Endosc 2006;64(2):263–7.
23. Song HY, Park SI, Jung HY, et al. Benign and malignant esophageal strictures: treatment with a polyurethane-covered retrievable expandable metallic stent. Radiology 1997;203(3):747–52.
24. Song HY, Jung HY, Park SI, et al. Covered retrievable expandable nitinol stents in patients with benign esophageal strictures: initial experience. Radiology 2000; 217(2):551–7.
25. Lakhtakia S. Refractory benign esophageal strictures: continuous, non-permanent dilation with a self-expandable metal esophageal stent [abstract]. Gastrointest Endosc 2007;65:284.
26. Eloubeidi MA, Lopes TL. Novel removable internally fully covered self-expanding metal esophageal stent: feasibility, technique of removal, and tissue response in humans. Am J Gastroenterol 2009;104(6):1374–81.
27. Bakken J, Song L, de Groan P, et al. Use of a fully covered self-expandable metal stent for the treatment of benign esophageal diseases. Gastrointest Endosc 2010;72(4):712–20.
28. Senousy BE, Gupte AR, Draganov PV, et al. Fully covered Alimaxx esophageal metal stents in the endoscopic treatment of benign esophageal diseases. Dig Dis Sci 2010;55(12):3399–403.
29. Repici A, Conio M, De Angelis C, et al. Temporary placement of an expandable polyester silicone-covered stent for treatment of refractory benign esophageal strictures. Gastrointest Endosc 2004;60(4):513–9.
30. Evrard S, Le Moine O, Lazaraki G, et al. Self-expanding plastic stents for benign esophageal lesions. Gastrointest Endosc 2004;60(6):894–900.
31. Holm AN, de la Mora Levy JG, Gostout CJ, et al. Self-expanding plastic stents in treatment of benign esophageal conditions. Gastrointest Endosc 2008;67(1): 20–5.

32. Triester SL, Fleischer DE, Sharma VK. Failure of self-expanding plastic stents in treatment of refractory benign esophageal strictures. Endoscopy 2006;38(5): 533–7.

33. Barthel JS, Kelley ST, Klapman JB. Management of persistent gastroesophageal anastomotic strictures with removable self-expandable polyester silicon-covered (Polyflex) stents: an alternative to serial dilation. Gastrointest Endosc 2008;67(3): 546–52.

34. Garcia-Cano J. Dilation of benign strictures in the esophagus and colon with the polyflex stent: a case series study. Dig Dis Sci 2008;53(2):341–6.

35. Pennathur A, Chang AC, McGrath KM, et al. Polyflex expandable stents in the treatment of esophageal disease: initial experience. Ann Thorac Surg 2008;85(6):1968–72 [discussion: 1973].

36. Dua KS, Vleggaar FP, Santharam R, et al. Removable self-expanding plastic esophageal stent as a continuous, non-permanent dilator in treating refractory benign esophageal strictures: a prospective two-center study. Am J Gastroenterol 2008;103(12):2988–94.

37. Oh YS, Kochman ML, Ahmad NA. Clinical outcomes after self-expanding plastic stent placement for refractory benign esophageal strictures. Dig Dis Sci 2010;55: 1344–8.

38. Repici A, Hassan C, Sharma P, et al. Systematic review: the role of self-expanding plastic stents for benign oesophageal strictures. Aliment Pharmacol Ther 2010; 31(12):1268–75.

39. Saito Y, Tanaka T, Andoh A, et al. Usefulness of biodegradable stents constructed of poly-l-lactic acid monofilaments in patients with benign esophageal stenosis. World J Gastroenterol 2007;13(29):3977–80.

40. Saito Y, Tanaka T, Andoh A, et al. Novel biodegradable stents for benign esophageal strictures following endoscopic submucosal dissection. Dig Dis Sci 2008; 53(2):330–3.

41. Dhar A, Johns E, O'Neill D. Biodegradable stents in refractory benign oesophageal strictures - first report of 4 patients from UK. Gastrointest Endosc 2009;69:M1487.

42. Repici A, Vleggaar FP, Hassan C, et al. Efficacy and safety of biodegradable stents for refractory benign esophageal strictures: the BEST (Biodegradable Esophageal Stent) study. Gastrointest Endosc 2010;72(5):927–34.

43. Jung GE, Sauer P, Schaible A. Tracheoesophageal fistula following implantation of a biodegradable stent for a refractory benign esophageal stricture. Endoscopy 2010;42(Suppl 2):E338–9.

44. Hair CS, Devonshire DA. Severe hyperplastic tissue stenosis of a novel biodegradable esophageal stent and subsequent successful management with high-pressure balloon dilation. Endoscopy 2010;42(Suppl 2):E132–3.

45. Brinster CJ, Singhal S, Lee L, et al. Evolving options in the management of esophageal perforation. Ann Thorac Surg 2004;77(4):1475–83.

46. Bufkin BL, Miller JI Jr, Mansour KA. Esophageal perforation: emphasis on management. Ann Thorac Surg 1996;61(5):1447–51 [discussion: 1451–2].

47. Zwischenberger JB, Savage C, Bidani A. Surgical aspects of esophageal disease: perforation and caustic injury. Am J Respir Crit Care Med 2002; 165(8):1037–40.

48. Attar S, Hankins JR, Suter CM, et al. Esophageal perforation: a therapeutic challenge. Ann Thorac Surg 1990;50(1):45–9 [discussion: 50–1].

49. Raju GS, Thompson C, Zwischenberger JB. Emerging endoscopic options in the management of esophageal leaks (video). Gastrointest Endosc 2005;62(2): 278–86.

50. Hermansson M, Johansson J, Gudbjartsson T, et al. Esophageal perforation in South of Sweden: results of surgical treatment in 125 consecutive patients. BMC Surg 2010;10:31.

51. Hirdes MM, Vleggaar FP, Van der Linde K, et al. Esophageal perforation due to removal of partially covered self-expanding metal stents placed for a benign perforation or leak. Endoscopy 2011;43(2):156–9.

52. Doniec JM, Schniewind B, Kahlke V, et al. Therapy of anastomotic leaks by means of covered self-expanding metallic stents after esophagogastrectomy. Endoscopy 2003;35(8):652–8.

53. Freeman RK, Van Woerkom JM, Ascioti AJ. Esophageal stent placement for the treatment of iatrogenic intrathoracic esophageal perforation. Ann Thorac Surg 2007;83(6):2003–7 [discussion: 2007–8].

54. Fukumoto R, Orlina J, McGinty J, et al. Use of Polyflex stents in treatment of acute esophageal and gastric leaks after bariatric surgery. Surg Obes Relat Dis 2007; 3(1):68–71 [discussion: 71–2].

55. Karbowski M, Schembre D, Kozarek R, et al. Polyflex self-expanding, removable plastic stents: assessment of treatment efficacy and safety in a variety of benign and malignant conditions of the esophagus. Surg Endosc 2008;22(5):1326–33.

56. Ott C, Ratiu N, Endlicher E, et al. Self-expanding Polyflex plastic stents in esophageal disease: various indications, complications, and outcomes. Surg Endosc 2007;21(6):889–96.

57. Siersema PD, Homs MY, Haringsma J, et al. Use of large-diameter metallic stents to seal traumatic nonmalignant perforations of the esophagus. Gastrointest Endosc 2003;58(3):356–61.

58. van Heel NC, Haringsma J, Spaander MC, et al. Short-term esophageal stenting in the management of benign perforations. Am J Gastroenterol 2010;105(7): 1515–20.

59. Johnsson E, Lundell L, Liedman B. Sealing of esophageal perforation or ruptures with expandable metallic stents: a prospective controlled study on treatment efficacy and limitations. Dis Esophagus 2005;18(4):262–6.

60. Petruzziello L, Tringali A, Riccioni ME, et al. Successful early treatment of Boerhaave's syndrome by endoscopic placement of a temporary self-expandable plastic stent without fluoroscopy. Gastrointest Endosc 2003;58(4):608–12.

61. vanBoeckel P, Dua K, Schmits R, et al. Covered self-expandable stents for the treatment of benign esophageal perforations and anastomotic leaks. Gastrointest Endosc 2010;71:313–4.

62. Chung MG, Kang DH, Park DK, et al. Successful treatment of Boerhaave's syndrome with endoscopic insertion of a self-expandable metallic stent: report of three cases and a review of the literature. Endoscopy 2001;33(10):894–7.

63. Langer FB, Wenzl E, Prager G, et al. Management of postoperative esophageal leaks with the Polyflex self-expanding covered plastic stent. Ann Thorac Surg 2005;79(2):398–403 [discussion: 404].

64. Schubert D, Scheidbach H, Kuhn R, et al. Endoscopic treatment of thoracic esophageal anastomotic leaks by using silicone-covered, self-expanding polyester stents. Gastrointest Endosc 2005;61(7):891–6.

65. Chak A, Singh R, Linden PA. Cove red stents for the treatment of life-threatening cervical esophageal anastomotic leaks. J Thorac Cardiovasc Surg 2011;141(3): 843–4.

66. Dai Y, S Chopra S, Kneif S. Management of esophageal anastomotic leaks, perforations, and fistulae with self-expanding plastic stents. J Thorac Cardiovasc Surg 2011;141:1213–7.

67. Eleftheriadis E, Kotzampassi K. Temporary stenting of acquired benign tracheoe-sophageal fistulas in critically ill ventilated patients. Surg Endosc 2005;19(6): 811–5.
68. Li YD, Tang GY, Cheng YS, et al. 13-year follow-up of a prospective comparison of the long-term clinical efficacy of temporary self-expanding metallic stents and pneumatic dilatation for the treatment of achalasia in 120 patients. AJR Am J Roentgenol 2010;195(6):1429–37.
69. Cheng YS, Ma F, Li YD, et al. Temporary self-expanding metallic stents for acha-lasia: a prospective study with a long-term follow-up. World J Gastroenterol 2010; 16(40):5111–7.
70. Li YD, Cheng YS, Li MH, et al. Temporary self-expanding metallic stents and pneumatic dilation for the treatment of achalasia: a prospective study with a long-term follow-up. Dis Esophagus 2010;23(5):361–7.
71. Zhu YQ, Cheng YS, Tang GY, et al. Comparison of temporary stent insertion with pneumatic dilation of the same diameter in the treatment of achalasia patients: a retrospective study. J Gastroenterol Hepatol 2010;25(3):499–505.
72. Zhu YQ, Cheng YS, Li F, et al. Application of the newly developed stents in the treatment of benign cardia stricture: an experimental comparative study. Gastro-intest Endosc 2011;73(2):329–37.
73. Wright G, Lewis H, Hogan B, et al. A self-expanding metal stent for complicated variceal hemorrhage: experience at a single center. Gastrointest Endosc 2010; 71(1):71–8.
74. Mishin I, Ghidirim G, Dolghii A, et al. Implantation of self-expanding metal stent in the treatment of severe bleeding from esophageal ulcer after endoscopic band ligation. Dis Esophagus 2010;23(7):E35–8.
75. Chan AC, Shin FG, Lam YH, et al. A comparison study on physical properties of self-expandable esophageal metal stents. Gastrointest Endosc 1999;49(4 Pt 1): 462–5.
76. Dua KS, Kozarek R, Kim J, et al. Self-expanding metal esophageal stent with anti-reflux mechanism. Gastrointest Endosc 2001;53(6):603–13.
77. Homs MY, Wahab PJ, Kuipers EJ, et al. Esophageal stents with antireflux valve for tumors of the distal esophagus and gastric cardia: a randomized trial. Gastroint-est Endosc 2004;60(5):695–702.
78. Laasch HU. Valved esophageal stents: benefits for patients outweigh perceived risks. Gastrointest Endosc 2005;62(5):822–3 [author reply: 823].
79. Laasch HU, Marriott A, Wilbraham L, et al. Effectiveness of open versus antireflux stents for palliation of distal esophageal carcinoma and prevention of symptom-atic gastroesophageal reflux. Radiology 2002;225(2):359–65.
80. Shim CS, Cho YD, Moon JH, et al. Fixation of a modified covered esophageal stent: its clinical usefulness for preventing stent migration. Endoscopy 2001; 33(10):843–8.
81. Hirdes MM, Siersema PD, Houben MH, et al. Stent-in-stent technique for removal of embedded esophageal self-expanding metal stents. Am J Gastroenterol 2011; 106:286–93.

Expandable Stents for Malignant Esophageal Disease

F.P. Vleggaar, MD, PhD*, P.D. Siersema, MD, PhD

KEYWORDS

• Esophagus • Cancer • Expandable • Stent • Dysphagia

Esophageal cancer (**Fig. 1**) is diagnosed in about 400,000 patients each year world-wide, and its incidence, particularly that of adenocarcinoma in the Western world, is increasing faster than that of any other malignancy.[1] This increasing incidence makes it the ninth most common malignancy and sixth on the list of cancer mortality causes. Notwithstanding recent progress in surgical and oncological treatment, most patients with esophageal cancer (50%–60%) present at a stage that is too advanced for cura-tive therapy, with many patients dying within a few months. Treatment of dysphagia is the main goal of palliative care in more than 50% of these incurable cases. Although many different palliative options for malignant dysphagia, such as radiotherapy,[2] laser,[3] argon plasma coagulation, photodynamic therapy,[4] local injection of alcohol,[5] or chemotherapeutic agents,[6] are available, expandable stent placement is the most commonly performed treatment modality worldwide because the above-mentioned options are less efficacious, more frequently associated with complications, or logis-tically more challenging.

ESOPHAGEAL CANCER

Rapid and persistent palliation of dysphagia is one of the main challenges in treating patients with incurable esophageal cancer to improve their quality of life. Brachyther-apy and placement of an expandable stent are the 2 most evidence-based palliative treatment options for these patients. Two randomized controlled studies comparing expandable stent placement with brachytherapy have shown that self-expandable metal stent (SEMS) insertion provides rapid palliation of dysphagia when compared with brachytherapy.[7,8] This difference in efficacy diminishes gradually over time, and brachytherapy seems to provide better relief of dysphagia after 3 months of

The authors have nothing to disclose.

Department of Gastroenterology and Hepatology, University Medical Center Utrecht, PO Box 85500, 3508 GA, Utrecht, The Netherlands
* Corresponding author. Department of Gastroenterology and Hepatology, University Medical Center Utrecht, Heidelberglaan 100, 3584 CX, Utrecht, The Netherlands.
E-mail address: f.vleggaar@umcutrecht.nl

Gastrointest Endoscopy Clin N Am 21 (2011) 377–388
doi:10.1016/j.giec.2011.04.006
1052-5157/11/$ – see front matter © 2011 Elsevier Inc. All rights reserved.

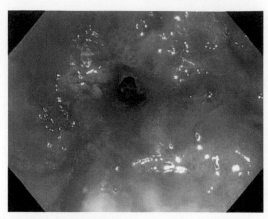

Fig. 1. Distal esophageal adenocarcinoma.

follow-up. However, in the study by Homs and colleagues,[7] the positive long-term outcome of brachytherapy was found in an intention-to-treat analysis, taking into account that 45 of the 101 patients allocated to brachytherapy also received a SEMS during follow-up for recurrent (**Fig. 2**) or persistent dysphagia, whereas only 2 of the 108 patients allocated to SEMS placement received additional brachytherapy. The long-term more-beneficial effect of brachytherapy may therefore be explained partly by additional SEMS placement during follow-up because of a lack of brachytherapy effect.

A broad array of expandable stent types is available to palliate malignant dysphagia (**Fig. 3**). The availability of so many different expandable stent designs attests to the fact that not one of the stents used today is significantly superior in all aspects to the others. However, one stent design does not fit all patients, and each stent type has specific features, which are advantageous or disadvantageous for stenting esophageal cancer (**Table 1**).

At present, 2 main categories of expandable stents are being used, such as SEMSs, which can be partially or fully covered, and self-expandable plastic stents (SEPSs). The most commonly used modern SEMSs in the Western world, such as the Ultraflex

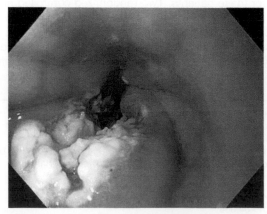

Fig. 2. Recurrent esophageal cancer after prior brachytherapy.

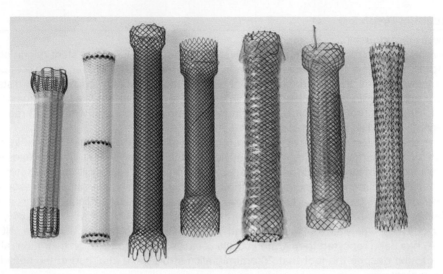

Fig. 3. Spectrum of expandable esophageal stents. From left to right: partially covered Ultraflex stent, Polyflex stent, partially covered Wallflex stent, partially covered Evolution stent, fully covered SX-Ella stent, fully covered Niti-S antimigration stent, and fully covered Alimaxx-E stent.

(Boston Scientific, Natick, MA, USA), Wallflex (Boston Scientific), Evolution (Cook Ireland Ltd, Limerick, Ireland), and Niti-S (Taewoong-Medical Co Ltd, Seoul, Korea) stents, are made of single or multiple braided nitinol wires with a silicone or polyurethane covering. The only commercially available SEPS (Polyflex stent, Boston Scientific) is built of a monofilament polyester infrastructure with a complete silicone cover. Rapid palliation of dysphagia, resulting in a decrease of the dysphagia score from 3 (able to swallow liquids) to 1 (occasional dysphagia for some solid food), is observed after placement of all the above-mentioned expandable stent types.

One of the main drawbacks in the palliation of malignant dysphagia with expandable stents is the occurrence of recurrent dysphagia because of stent migration, tumoral and nontumoral tissue ingrowth or overgrowth, or food impaction. Prevention of these stent-related complications remains one of the major challenges for developing new stent designs.

Table 1
Advantages and disadvantages of the different stent types used for treating malignant dysphagia caused by esophageal cancer

Stent Type	Advantage	Disadvantage
Partially covered SEMS	Low migration risk	Tissue ingrowth or overgrowth at stent ends Removal may be difficult
Fully covered SEMS	Safe and easy removal Low risk of tissue ingrowth	High migration risk Tissue hyperplasia at stent ends
SEPS	Safe and easy removal Low rate of hyperplastic overgrowth at stent ends No tissue ingrowth	High migration risk Complex and stiff/large introducer system

Recurrent Dysphagia

Stent migration

Several stent- and patient-related factors are known risk factors for stent migration, leading to recurrent dysphagia. Migration is more frequently observed when a stent is placed across the gastroesophageal (GE) junction, probably because the distal stent end projects freely in the gastric lumen and is therefore not fixed to the gastric wall. Regression of tumor volume because of concurrent chemotherapy and radiotherapy is another cause of stent migration.[9]

In general, migration rates of fully covered stents, either SEMSs or SEPSs, are higher than those of partially covered stents. Embedding of the uncovered stent ends leads to better fixation of the stent to the esophageal wall. The advantage of fully covered stents is that it allows removal if indicated, although this is rarely needed in incurable esophageal cancer. Studies on partially covered stents, such as the Ultraflex, Evolution, and Wallflex stents, have shown migration rates of 4% to 23%,[7,10–15] 5%,[16] and 6%,[17] respectively, whereas the fully covered Alimaxx-E stent (Alveolus, Charlotte, NC, USA) has been reported to migrate in 36% of cases.[18] This rather high migration rate was found despite the fact that 20 antimigration struts were attached to the outside of the stent.

In the previous 5 years, many other antimigration modifications to the design of esophageal fully covered expandable stents have been developed (**Table 2**). The SX-Ella stent (Ella-CS, Hradec Kralove, Czech Republic) has an antimigration ring circumferentially attached to the proximal portion of the stent. This ring not only functions as a circular hook preventing migration but also has a mechanism that reduces risk of injury to the esophageal wall with excessive traction. The stent flares to 25 mm at its proximal and distal ends and has a midbody diameter of 20 mm. Uitdehaag and colleagues[19] treated 44 patients with the SX-Ella stent and found improvement in the dysphagia score form 3 to 1. However, stent migration leading to recurrent dysphagia was observed in 14% to 20% of patients, suggesting that the antimigration ring and flares are not sufficient in preventing migration. Moreover, hemorrhage (25%) and fistula formation (6%) were frequently observed with this stent type. The investigators hypothesized that these complications might have been caused by friction of the antimigration ring resulting in esophageal wall injury.

The fully covered Niti-S antimigration stent (Taewoong Medical Co Ltd) has a double-layer configuration over its entire length, consisting of an inner polyurethane layer and an outer uncovered nitinol mesh, which allows stent embedding to prevent migration. Relatively large flares of 26 mm at both ends are a second antimigration feature of this stent design. Verschuur and colleagues[10] performed a randomized trial (n = 125 patients) comparing the Niti-S stent with the Ultraflex and Polyflex stents. Although these 3 stent designs were equally effective and safe for palliation of malignant dysphagia, stent migration was most frequently seen with the Polyflex stent

| Table 2 | | |
Efficacy of antimigration modifications to expandable stents		
Stent Modification	**Efficacy**	**Drawback**
Small struts on the outside	−	None
Antimigration collar	+/−	Hemorrhage/fistula
Outer uncovered mesh	+/−	Inability to remove
Large-diameter stent/flares	+	Hemorrhage/perforation/fistula

Abbreviations: −, not effective; +/−, modestly effective; +, effective.

(29%). The Ultraflex and double-layer Niti-S stents had similar stent migration rates of 17% and 12%, respectively.

Large-diameter expandable stents were introduced to reduce the risk of migration, which is because of an increased expansile pressure on the esophageal wall. An analysis of a large database of 338 patients treated with 3 types of stents (Ultraflex, Flamingo Wallstent [Boston Scientific], or Gianturco Z-stent [Cook Ireland Ltd]) with small or large diameters showed that large-diameter stents reduce the risk of recurrent dysphagia from stent migration, tissue overgrowth, or food obstruction (adjusted hazard ratio, 0.35; 95% confidence interval [CI], 0.2–0.7).[15] The downside of placement of a wide-body stent, however, was the increased risk of stent-related complications, such as hemorrhage, perforation, fistula, and fever, which was particularly true for the wide-body Gianturco Z-stent (adjusted hazard ratio, 5.0; 95% CI, 1.3–19.1).

If the stent migrates to the stomach or bowel, the authors advise stent removal, preferably endoscopically, to prevent further injury to the gastrointestinal tract. Complications caused by migrated expandable esophageal stents, such as small bowel obstruction[20,21] or perforation[22] and formation of a gastropleural fistula,[23] have been reported. The authors' own (F.P.V. and P.D.S., unpublished data, 2011) experience is similar to these findings.

Tumoral or nontumoral tissue ingrowth or overgrowth

Stent occlusion because of ingrowth of tissue through the uncovered mesh or overgrowth at the stent ends is another cause of recurrent dysphagia. The incidence of tissue ingrowth and overgrowth at uncovered stent ends varies from 3% to 31% in series using the Ultraflex stent,[7,10,12–15] whereas it was reported in 14% and 10% of cases after placement of the partially covered Evolution and Wallflex stents, respectively.[16,17] The risk of developing stent occlusion because of reactive tissue growth increases with longer dwell times. Radial force and diameter of the stent as well as the nitinol or metal material of the stent seem to be the other factors causing reactive tissue ingrowth and overgrowth.

Tissue ingrowth and, to some extent, overgrowth is thought to be reduced with fully covered stents, although overgrowth has been reported in 10% to 30% of cases with a fully covered Alimaxx-E stent[18] and in 5% to 24% of cases treated with a Niti-S stent.[24] The risk of developing tumoral overgrowth can be reduced by using stents that are substantially longer than the malignant stricture.

Fully covered SEPSs, with the Polyflex being the only stent that is commercially available, induce less-reactive nontumoral tissue growth. Verschuur and colleagues[10] showed that tissue ingrowth or overgrowth occurred more frequently with partially covered Ultraflex stents (31%) than with Polyflex stents (10%) or fully covered Niti-S stents (24%). This cause of recurrent dysphagia was observed after a median of 79 days after stent placement and treated by placement of a second stent. However, a randomized study by Conio and colleagues[12] that compared the Ultraflex stent with the Polyflex stent did not show a difference in hyperplastic tissue reaction.

The Polyflex stent has some features that might increase the risk of esophageal perforation. The applicator, in which the stent is loaded before placement, has a diameter of 12 to 14 mm depending on stent size, and is rather rigid. In addition, the dilator at the tip of the introducer system is short, which may complicate its passage across angulated strictures because of inappropriate transmission of force. Another drawback of the Polyflex stent is its known relatively high migration rate, particularly in cases with distal stenoses. This is a significant problem. Migration rates range from 13% to 29% in randomized studies comparing SEPSs with SEMSs in patients with unresectable esophageal cancer.[25]

Food obstruction

Food impaction within the stent is yet another cause of recurrent dysphagia. The incidence of this complication varies, but with the latest versions of stents, such as the Evolution and Wallflex, symptomatic food impaction was observed in just 7% and 5% of patients, respectively.[16,17] This low frequency may be because of the smooth silicone covering on the inside of these stents, which facilitates food passage through the stent. To reduce the risk of this complication, patients should be advised to chew thoroughly and to drink, preferably carbonated beverages, during and after a meal.

Pain

The rate of retrosternal pain after stent placement seems to vary depending on the type of stent used. A relatively high frequency of retrosternal pain was observed after placement of partially covered Wallflex (31%)[17] and Alimaxx-E stents (22%).[18] In contrast, pain was less frequently observed after placement of an Evolution stent (9%),[16] Ultraflex stent (6%–7%),[10,11] Choostent (MI Tech Co Ltd, Seoul, Korea, 3%),[11] and Niti-S stent (10%–12%).[10,24] Increased expansion force and decreased flexibility of some stent types may play a role in inducing retrosternal pain. Because it has been demonstrated that previous radiation and/or chemotherapy is associated with a higher risk of retrosternal pain after stent placement,[17,26] the above-mentioned pain rates may be because of potential bias. The authors advise prescribing opiates when there is retrosternal pain after expandable stent placement.

GE reflux

Stent placement across the GE junction may lead to reflux of gastric contents in some patients because a stent in this position prevents the lower esophageal sphincter to function. These patients are best treated with high-dose proton pump inhibitors (PPIs); however, in some patients, reflux symptoms persist despite treatment with PPIs. These patients may be candidates for an antireflux stent.

Several antireflux stent designs have been evaluated in randomized trials.[27–31] Placement of a Z-stent (Cook Medical Inc, Limerick, Ireland) with a windsocklike valve on the distal end to prevent GE reflux was found to significantly reduce reflux symptoms compared with the standard open stents, but more objective data, such as pH measurement, were not obtained.[28] The Fer-X Ella stent (Ella-CS) actually resulted in increased reflux symptoms and total acid exposure time in the antireflux stent group compared with the open stent group.[27] Inadequate valve characteristics, such as a relatively short length of the windsock valve and the floppy material used, were thought to be the underlying causes of this surprising outcome. To further evaluate antireflux stents, a Korean study group compared the Do stent (MI Tech Co Ltd) that has a tricuspid antireflux valve, another antireflux stent with an S-shaped valve and long leaflets (MI Tech Co Ltd), and a standard open stent (MI Tech).[31] The S-shaped valve significantly reduced reflux symptoms and total acid exposure time compared with the open and Do stents.

Given the conflicting results in different studies with different stent designs, the authors do not recommend the routine use of antireflux stents in patients with distal esophageal or gastric cardia cancer.

ESOPHAGORESPIRATORY FISTULAS

Malignant esophagorespiratory fistulas (EFs) (**Fig. 4**) are a complication of primary tumor growth or recurrence of esophageal or lung cancer, or may result from chemotherapy and/or radiation therapy, leading to tumor necrosis. EFs result in frequent

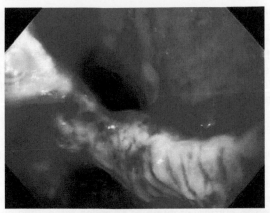

Fig. 4. A large EF. Lower lumen is the esophageal lumen and the upper lumen is the fistula.

aspiration (pneumonia) and poor nutritional intake. The mean survival of patients with this complication is from 1 to 6 weeks with supportive care alone.[32]

Surgical closure, resection, or bypass surgery does not produce good palliative results for this patient population because of high morbidity and mortality. Various studies on the use of (partially) covered SEMSs for malignant fistulas have reported successful fistula closure in 87% to 91% of patients (**Fig. 5**).[33–35] Ross and colleagues[33] reported symptom improvement in 90% of patients with EFs treated with SEMS placement. SEMSs can also be placed in the trachea or bronchus to close the fistulae. Furthermore, combined airway and esophageal stenting should be considered, particularly when the stent in 1 location (tracheal or esophagus) does not seal the fistula. In addition, because stent placement in the esophagus may cause compression on the airways, particularly the trachea, stenting both the esophagus and the airway may be needed. Randomized studies comparing different stent designs and stenting options are not available.

Recently, Herth and colleagues[36] published their experience with esophageal (n = 37), airway (n = 65), or combined esophageal and airway stent placement

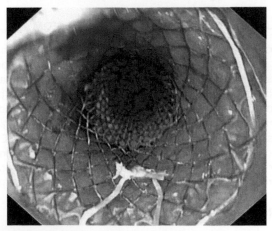

Fig. 5. Endoscopic photograph of a partially covered Wallflex stent placed for sealing a malignant esophagorespiratory fistula.

(n = 10) in 112 patients with malignant fistulas, of which 74% had advanced lung cancer. Initial closure of the fistula was achieved in all patients.[36] Survival was lower in the airway stent group (219 days; 95% CI, 197–241) than in the esophageal stent (263 days; 95% CI, 244–281) or combined stent (253 days; 95% CI, 193–313) groups. In addition to the site of stent placement, localization of the fistula in the airway was another independent risk factor, with the trachea, carina, and left main bronchus giving more favorable results than the right main bronchus.

BRIDGE-TO-SURGERY STENTING

An increasing proportion of patients with resectable esophageal cancer are being treated with neoadjuvant chemotherapy and radiotherapy or definite chemoradiation. Some of these patients into, however, have severe dysphagia and weight loss while receiving such treatment. Temporary expandable stent placement, sometimes referred to as bridge-to-surgery stenting, is an option rather than nasoenteric feeding tube or percutaneous endoscopic gastrostomy tube placement and instantly restores esophageal patency, leading to improvement of food intake.

To date, a total of 104 patients with curable esophageal cancer have been treated with temporary removable expandable stent placement before starting neoadjuvant therapy. Of these, 36 patients received a (partially) covered SEMS and 68 patients received a Polyflex stent.[9,37–41] Instant relief of dysphagia after successful stent placement was achieved in more than 97% of these patients. In a nonrandomized study, Siddiqui and colleagues[39] showed that improvement of nutritional status was comparable between patients who received jejunostomy feeding and those who received a temporary esophageal expandable stent.

Stent migration occurred in 18% to 48% of patients in studies that included more than 10 patients. Regression of the tumor volume in response to treatment and the stent design, such as a SEPS or a fully covered SEMS, likely account for these high migration rates.[9,37,39–41] Other major complications in these 104 patients included development of an EF in 3 cases (3%), esophageal perforation in 1 case, jejunal perforation due to stent migration in 1 case, mediastinitis in 1 case, and bleeding in 1 case. Most stents were uneventfully removed by endoscopic means before esophagectomy. Nevertheless, it remains to be seen whether a major complication rate of 7% can be justified in a patient group with potentially curable esophageal cancer.

RECURRENT LOCAL TUMOR GROWTH AFTER ESOPHAGECTOMY

A substantial proportion of patients present with recurrent dysphagia because of locoregional recurrence or mediastinal metastasis within 2 years after esophagectomy and gastric conduit reconstruction (**Fig. 6**). Because the prognosis is dismal in these patients and rapid relief of dysphagia is therefore required, expandable stent placement seems the most optimal palliative treatment option. A recent prospective cohort study on 81 patients with recurrent tumor growth after esophagectomy (dysphagia, n = 66; fistula, n = 15) showed restoration of luminal patency in 98% of cases after SEMS placement.[42] Recurrent dysphagia after stent placement because of migration, food obstruction, or tissue ingrowth or overgrowth was observed in 27% of patients and was managed endoscopically. Previously published smaller series have shown comparable results.

EXTRINSIC MALIGNANT COMPRESSION ON THE ESOPHAGUS

Malignant dysphagia because of extrinsic compression on the esophagus is another indication for palliative expandable stent placement because the majority of these

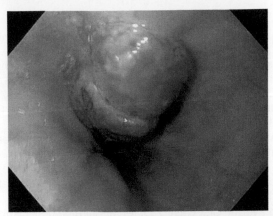

Fig. 6. Recurrent cancer at the anastomosis after esophagectomy for esophageal cancer.

patients are incurable, with a predicted life expectancy of less than 6 months. Partially as well as fully covered SEMSs have been used in this patient population with good relief of dysphagia. Despite the absence of intraluminal tumor growth, stent migration was observed in only 4% of cases in a recently published series of 50 patients, although a relatively short median survival of 44 days may have led to underestimation of this complication.[43]

VERY PROXIMAL ESOPHAGEAL CANCERS

Tumors close to (<2 cm) the upper esophageal sphincter (UES) are seen in 7% to 10% of all esophageal cancers and are traditionally considered to be a contraindication to expandable stent placement because of the increased risk of complications such as perforation, airway compression, proximal migration, aspiration pneumonia, and discomfort due to pain and globus sensation. However, this belief has changed because several studies have shown that stent placement in patients with tumors located close to the UES can be safe and effective.[44,45] Compression on the airway caused by the stent can be prevented by using small-diameter stents (10–16 mm) or with stenting of the trachea before esophageal stent placement. Furthermore, many of these patients have decreased sensitivity for a foreign body because of previous local radiotherapy or surgery.

SUMMARY

The currently available expandable stents for malignant esophageal disease provide rapid and sufficient palliation of dysphagia. The rate of recurrent dysphagia due to stent migration varies, with SEPSs and fully covered SEMSs having higher migration rates than partially covered SEMSs. In contrast, tissue ingrowth or overgrowth is more frequently observed with partially covered stents. Antireflux stents can be used in patients with refractory reflux esophagitis despite PPI treatment; however, reported results are conflicting. Placement of expandable stents also offers adequate palliation for patients with EFs, extrinsic malignant compression, local tumor recurrence after esophagectomy, and very proximal esophageal cancer and is currently an option as bridge to surgery.

REFERENCES

1. Siersema PD. Esophageal cancer. Gastroenterol Clin North Am 2008;37: 943–64.
2. Homs MY, Eijkenboom WM, Siersema PD. Single-dose brachytherapy for the palliative treatment of esophageal cancer. Endoscopy 2005;37:1143–8.
3. Fleischer D, Sivak MV Jr. Endoscopic Nd: YAG laser therapy as palliation for esophagogastric cancer. Parameters affecting initial outcome. Gastroenterology 1985;89:827–31.
4. Okunaka T, Kato H, Conaka C, et al. Photodynamic therapy for esophageal carcinoma. Surg Endosc 1990;4:150–3.
5. Wadleigh RG, Abbasi S, Korman L. Palliative ethanol injection of unresectable advanced esophageal carcinoma combined with chemoradiation. Am J Med Sci 2006;331:110–2.
6. Burris HA 3rd, Vogel CL, Castro D, et al. Intratumoral cisplatin/epinephrine-injectable gel as a palliative treatment for accessible solid tumors: a multicenter pilot study. Otolaryngol Head Neck Surg 1998;118:496–503.
7. Homs MY, Steyerberg EW, Eijkenboom WM, et al. Single-dose brachytherapy versus metal stent placement for the palliation of dysphagia from oesophageal cancer: multicentre randomised trial. Lancet 2004;364:1497–504.
8. Bergquist H, Wenger U, Johnsson E, et al. Stent insertion or endoluminal brachytherapy as palliation of patients with advanced cancer of the esophagus and gastroesophageal junction. Results of a randomized, controlled clinical trial. Dis Esophagus 2005;18:131–9.
9. Adler DG, Fang J, Wong R, et al. Placement of Polyflex stents in patients with locally advanced esophageal cancer is safe and improves dysphagia during neoadjuvant therapy. Gastrointest Endosc 2009;70:614–9.
10. Verschuur EM, Repici A, Kuipers EJ, et al. New design esophageal stents for the palliation of dysphagia from esophageal or gastric cancer cardia cancer: a randomized trial. Am J Gastroenterol 2008;103:304–12.
11. Bona D, Laface L, Bonavina L, et al. Covered nitinol stents for the treatment of esophageal strictures and leaks. World J Gastroenterol 2010;16:2260–4.
12. Conio M, Repici A, Battaglia G, et al. A randomized prospective comparison of self-expandable plastic stents and partially covered self-expandable metal stents in the palliation of malignant esophageal dysphagia. Am J Gastroenterol 2007; 102:2667–77.
13. Homs MY, Steyerberg EW, Kuipers EJ, et al. Causes and treatment of recurrent dysphagia after self-expanding metal stent placement for palliation of esophageal carcinoma. Endoscopy 2004;36:880–6.
14. Sabharwal T, Hamady MS, Chui S, et al. A randomized prospective comparison of the Flamingo Wallstent and Ultraflex stent for palliation of dysphagia associated with lower third esophageal carcinoma. Gut 2003;52:922–6.
15. Verschuur EM, Steyerberg EW, Kuipers EJ, et al. Effect of stent size on complications and recurrent dysphagia in patients with esophageal or gastric cardia cancer. Gastrointest Endosc 2007;65:592–601.
16. Van Boeckel PG, Repici A, Vleggaar FP, et al. A new metal stent with a controlled-release system for palliation of malignant dysphagia: a prospective, multicenter study. Gastrointest Endosc 2010;71:455–60.
17. Van Boeckel PG, Siersema PD, Sturgess R, et al. A new partially covered metal stent for palliation of malignant dysphagia: a prospective follow-up study. Gastrointest Endosc 2010;72:1269–73.

18. Uitdehaag MJ, van Hooft JE, Verschuur EM, et al. A fully-covered stent (Alimaxx-E) for the palliation of malignant dysphagia: a prospective follow-up study. Gastrointest Endosc 2009;70:1082–9.

19. Uitdehaag MJ, Siersema PD, Spaander MC, et al. A new fully covered stent with antimigration properties for the palliation of malignant dysphagia: a prospective cohort study. Gastrointest Endosc 2010;71:600–5.

20. Bay J, Penninga L. Small bowel ileus caused by migration of esophageal stent. Ugerskr Laeger 2010;172:2234–5 [in Danish].

21. Harries R, Campbell J, Ghosh S. Fractured migrated oesophageal stent fragment presenting as small bowel obstruction three years after insertion. Ann R Coll Surg Engl 2010;92:W14–5.

22. Reddy VM, Sutton CD, Miller AS. Terminal ileum perforation as a consequence of a migrated and fractured oesophageal stent. Case Rep Gastroenterol 2009;15:61–6.

23. Furlong H, Nasr A, Walsh TN. Gastropleural fistula: a complication of esophageal self-expanding metallic stent migration. Endoscopy 2009;41:E38–9.

24. Verschuur EM, Homs MY, Steyerberg EW, et al. A new esophageal stent design (Niti-S) for the prevention of migration: a prospective follow-up study in 42 patients. Gastrointest Endosc 2006;63:134–40.

25. Vleggaar FP. Stent placement in esophageal cancer as a bridge to surgery. Gastrointest Endosc 2009;70:620–2.

26. Homs MY, Hansen BE, van Blankenstein M, et al. Prior radiation and/or chemotherapy has no effect on the outcome of metal stent placement for oesophagogastric carcinoma. Eur J Gastroenterol Hepatol 2004;16:163–70.

27. Homs MY, Wahab PJ, Kuipers EJ, et al. Esophageal stents with antireflux valve for tumors of the distal esophagus and gastric cardia: a randomized trial. Gastrointest Endosc 2004;60:695–702.

28. Laasch HU, Marriott A, Wilbraham L, et al. Effectiveness of open versus antireflux stents for palliation of distal esophageal carcinoma and prevention of symptomatic gastroesophageal reflux. Radiology 2002;225:359–65.

29. Power C, Byrne PJ, Lim K, et al. Superiority of anti-reflux stent compared with conventional stents in the palliative management of patients with cancer of the lower esophagus and esophago-gastric junction: results of a randomized clinical trial. Dis Esophagus 2007;20:466–70.

30. Sabharwal T, Gulati MS, Fotiadis N, et al. Randomised comparison of the FerX Ella antireflux stent and the ultraflex stent: proton pump inhibitor combination for prevention of post-stent reflux in patients with esophageal carcinoma involving the esophago-gastric junction. J Gastroenterol Hepatol 2008;23:723–8.

31. Shim CS, Jung IS, Cheon YK, et al. Management of malignant stricture of the esophagogastric junction with a newly designed self-expanding metal stent with an antireflux mechanism. Endoscopy 2005;37:335–9.

32. Reed MF, Mathisen DJ. Tracheoesophageal fistula. Chest Surg Clin N Am 2003; 13:271–89.

33. Ross WA, Alkassab F, Lynch PM, et al. Evolving role of self-expanding metal stents in the treatment of malignant dysphagia and fistulas. Gastrointest Endosc 2007;65:70–6.

34. May A, Ell C. Palliative treatment of malignant esophagorespiratory fistulas with Gianturco-Z stents. A prospective clinical trial and review of the literature on covered metal stents. Am J Gastroenterol 1998;93:532–5.

35. Raijman I, Siddique I, Ajani J, et al. Palliation of malignant dysphagia and fistulae with coated expandable metal stents: experience with 101 patients. Gastrointest Endosc 1998;48:172–9.

36. Herth FJ, Peter S, Baty F, et al. Combined airway and oesophageal stenting in malignant airway-oesophageal fistulas: a prospective study. Eur Respir J 2010; 36:1370–4.
37. Bower M, Jones W, Vessels B, et al. Nutritional support with endoluminal stenting during neoadjuvant therapy for esophageal malignancy. Ann Surg Oncol 2009; 16:3161–8.
38. Martin R, Duvall R, Ellis S, et al. The use of self-expanding silicone stents in esophageal cancer care: optimal pre-, peri-, and postoperative car. Surg Endosc 2009;23:615–21.
39. Siddiqui AA, Glynn C, Loren D, et al. Self-expanding plastic esophageal stents versus jejunostomy tubes for the maintenance of nutrition during neoadjuvant chemoradiation therapy in patients with esophageal cancer: a retrospective study. Dis Esophagus 2009;22:216–22.
40. Lopes TL, Eloubeidi MA. A pilot study of fully covered self-expandable metal stents prior to neoadjuvant therapy for locally advanced esophageal cancer. Dis Esophagus 2010;23:309–15.
41. Langer FB, Schoppmann SF, Prager G, et al. Temporary placement of self-expanding oesophageal stents as bridging for neo-adjuvant therapy. Ann Surg Oncol 2010;17:470–5.
42. Van Heel NC, Haringsma J, Spaander MC, et al. Esophageal stents for the palliation of malignant dysphagia and fistula recurrence after esophagectomy. Gastrointest Endosc 2010;72:249–54.
43. Van Heel NC, Haringsma J, Spaander MC, et al. Esophageal stents for the relief of malignant dysphagia due to extrinsic compression. Endoscopy 2010;42:536–40.
44. Verschuur EM, Kuipers EJ, Siersema PD. Esophageal stents for malignant strictures close to the upper esophageal sphincter. Gastrointest Endosc 2007;66:1082–90.
45. Eleftheriadis E, Kotzampassi K. Endoprosthesis implantation at the pharyngo-esophageal level: problems, limitations and challenges. World J Gastroenterol 2006;12:2103–8.

Enteral Stents for Malignant Gastric Outlet Obstruction

Bryan Brimhall, MD, Douglas G. Adler, MD*

KEYWORDS

• Gastric outlet obstruction • Enteral stent • Gastrojejunostomy
• Malignancy

Malignant gastric outlet obstruction (GOO) is defined as the inability of the stomach to empty because of mechanical obstruction at the level of either the distal stomach or the proximal small bowel.[1] GOO is a late complication of a variety of cancers including pancreatic, gastric, duodenal, ampullary, cholangiocarcinoma, and metastatic carcinoma, with pancreatic cancer the most common cause.[1,2] An estimated 43,140 cases of pancreatic cancer and 21,000 cases of gastric cancer were diagnosed during the year 2010.[3,4] GOO occurs in approximately 15% to 20% of patients diagnosed with malignancies such as pancreatic cancer.[5–7] It has been reported that surgical options are unsuccessful in up to 85% of pancreatic malignancies and as many as 40% of patients with gastric cancer.[1,8,9] Clinical symptoms of GOO include severe nausea, intractable vomiting, abdominal pain, malnutrition, and dehydration.[7,10] These symptoms may be misinterpreted by clinicians as side effects of chemotherapy and radiation or simply as manifestations of advanced cancer.[1] Malignant GOO is frequently associated with unresectable disease. Once GOO is diagnosed, mean life expectancy ranges from 7 to 20 weeks.[2,11–14]

The classic palliative management for patients with GOO is open or laparoscopic gastrojejunostomy; however, the past decade has seen the introduction and widespread use of enteral stents to manage these patients.[15–17] The ability to use enteral stents as a palliative measure to alleviate symptomatic GOO provides an alternative to surgery and other approaches including enteral and parenteral nutrition. Enteral stent placement has also been shown to improve the quality of life in patients with GOO.[16,18–20]

This article reviews the etiology, evaluation, and treatment of malignant GOO with a focus on enteral stents.

Division of Gastroenterology and Hepatology, Department of Internal Medicine, University of Utah School of Medicine, Salt Lake City, UT 84132, USA
* Corresponding author. 30 North 1900 East 4R118, Salt Lake City, UT 84132.
E-mail address: douglas.adler@hsc.utah.edu

Gastrointest Endoscopy Clin N Am 21 (2011) 389–403
doi:10.1016/j.giec.2011.04.002
1052-5157/11/$ – see front matter © 2011 Elsevier Inc. All rights reserved.

TYPES OF CANCER ASSOCIATED WITH GOO

GOO is commonly encountered in the context of a variety of cancers including pancreatic, gastric, duodenal, ampullary, cholangiocarcinoma, hepatobiliary, metastatic, and recurrent malignancy following surgical resection.[15,18,21–23] One study involving 176 patients treated at 4 major centers over 7 years cited primary pancreatic malignancy as the most common reason for GOO, corroborating findings from other investigators. Gastric malignancies were the next most common reason for GOO.[24] Other studies have supported pancreatic malignancy as being the most common site to require and benefit from the use of an enteral stent, although some studies have had conflicting data, with gastric malignancy being the most common, followed by pancreatic malignancies.[7,25–27] Metastatic cancers to the bowel itself, such as colon cancer, bulky lesions, or adenopathy at the porta hepatis, are also common causes of GOO.[7] Duodenal, ampullary, cholangiocarcinoma, hepatobiliary, and recurrent malignancies are usually less common in incidence than either pancreatic or gastric malignancies, but have been repeatedly reported.[22,24,25]

SYMPTOMS AND DIAGNOSIS OF GOO

Symptoms of GOO include nausea, vomiting, weight loss, dehydration, hypoalbuminemia, jaundice, and the inability to tolerate oral intake.[1,7,10,17] Symptoms of GOO can overlap with symptoms of the primary malignancy and may be missed by clinicians, or be attributed to different treatments including chemotherapy and/or radiation.[1]

Diagnosis is based on history, physical examination, results of imaging studies, and findings at endoscopy. A history suggestive of vomiting undigested food hours after eating and nonbilious emesis is strongly suggestive of GOO: these findings imply that food cannot leave the stomach and that the second portion of the duodenum has been isolated from the proximal stomach, respectively.[1,28]

Physical examination in these patients can be of value, and one may elicit a succession splash on auscultation of the upper abdomen, similar to that seen in children with pyloric stenosis. This maneuver has a sensitivity of 48% if a splash is heard more than 3 hours following ingestion of food.[29]

Imaging techniques vary widely and include plain abdominal radiographs, ultrasonography, upper gastrointestinal (UGI) contrast studies, and abdominal computed tomography (CT). Plain films may show an enlarged gastric bubble, dilated proximal duodenum, and limited air in the small bowel. UGI contrast studies can be performed with either barium or water-soluble contrast. These tests will often demonstrate the location and severity of the site of obstruction, and can be particularly helpful if GOO is incomplete. CT studies may also show a distended stomach, dilated proximal duodenum, decompressed distal small bowel, and the obstructing lesion itself.

The gold standard for the diagnosis of GOO is endoscopy (**Fig. 1**). Endoscopy is not recommended until appropriate history, physical, and imaging studies are completed. Upper endoscopy can then be performed allowing direct visualization and assessment of severity, nature, site, and biopsy of the obstruction.[30] If the stricture can be traversed with the endoscope this is helpful, but in practice is rare. Fluoroscopy should be used to enhance visibility and safety during the entire procedure. Deployment of an enteral stent involves first traversing the stricture with a soft flexible guide wire. Some endoscopists prefer to then advance a catheter across the stricture and then exchange the soft wire for a stiffer guide wire, but there is no universally accepted preference for type of guide wire. The catheter can also be used to inject contrast across the stricture to fully delineate its length and geometry, which greatly aids in the

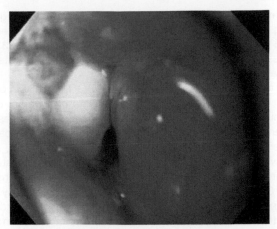

Fig. 1. Endoscopic image of gastric outlet obstruction (GOO) at the level of the apex of the duodenal bulb secondary to pancreatic cancer. Note the pinpoint lumen at the center of the image.

selection of the proper stent size with regard to both diameter and length. The catheter is then removed, leaving the guide wire in place across the stricture. The stent is then passed through the working channel of the endoscope over the guide wire, and deployed using both direct visualization and fluoroscopic assistance.[7,8,28,30] Most experts recommend the use of fluoroscopy even if the stricture can be traversed without difficulty.[12]

NONSTENT-BASED TREATMENTS FOR GOO

The classic palliative management of GOO has been either open or laparoscopic gastrojejunostomy (with or without concomitant biliary bypass). Other treatments such as radiation, chemotherapy, nasoenteric feeding tubes, gastric decompression tubes, and total parental nutrition have been used independently or in combination with enteral stent placement and/or gastrojejunostomy.[11,24,31,32]

Laparoscopic surgical gastrojejunostomy is an excellent option, and has been shown to reduce hospital stay and associated morbidity when compared with open gastrojejunostomy.[33] Unfortunately, many patients with GOO are poor surgical candidates because of their advanced underlying disease, poor nutritional status, and short life expectancy.[1] Gastrojejunostomy is performed by attaching a sufficient length of a loop of jejunum to the antecolic portion of the greater curvature of the stomach using a staple gun and/or suture.[20,34] If the patient has a concomitant biliary stricture, this can be treated via the creation of a surgical biliary bypass or a biliary stent placed endoscopically if the second portion of the duodenum is accessible beyond the site of the GOO. In one study of 23 patients undergoing open gastrojejunostomy, 15 were found to have a biliary stricture, 10 underwent surgical bypass, and 5 had a biliary stent placed endoscopically.[35]

Radiation therapy is also used in the treatment of malignant GOO. Studies investigating monotherapy with radiation have found an increased incidence of tumor growth and fibrosis with worsening obstruction. Mogavero and colleagues[36] found that GOO developed in 7 of 63 patients treated with radiation following curative resection or stent placement for cholangiocarcinoma. However, other studies have demonstrated clinical success with radiation therapy combined with enteral stent placement. In a study by Park and colleagues,[37] radiation therapy following enteral stent placement prolonged stent patency (odds ratio [OR] 0.221, 95% confidence interval [CI] 0.055–0.884, P = .033). By contrast, Im and colleagues[31] found no significant association between stent patency and radiation in 16 patients.

Chemotherapy is also used in the treatment of GOO, usually in combination with another treatment modality. There are conflicting data on whether chemotherapy is helpful in maintaining stent patency. In a study by Cho and colleagues[11] of 27 patients who received chemotherapy, stent patency was prolonged in comparison with those who did not receive chemotherapy (OR 0.34, 95% CI 0.13–0.91, P = .03). Other studies have shown similar results, with chemotherapy prolonging stent patency.[24,32] By contrast, Im and colleagues[31] found no association between chemotherapy and stent patency in 6 patients who received palliative chemotherapy. Chemotherapy following stent placement has also been associated with increased stent migration in comparison with no other palliative treatment or chemoradiation (42.9% vs 10% vs 9.1%, P = .042).[31]

Nasoenteric tubes are used to treat GOO when life expectancy is very short, typically days to a few weeks.[35] Nasoenteric tubes in patients with short life expectancies are often used as a comfort measure to provide hydration, sometimes in combination with percutaneous endoscopic gastrostomy tubes (for gastric decompression). Nasoenteric tubes should not be left for longer than 1 month.[38] If it is expected that the patient will survive longer than 1 month, enteral stent placement or gastrojejunostomy should be performed. A benefit seen with nasoenteric tubes includes the possibility of removal.

Total parental nutrition (TPN) is often used for the same reasons as nasoenteric tubes. TPN has been used as a temporizing measure before surgery to improve nutritional status through hydration, correction of electrolyte imbalances, improvement in serum albumin levels, and so forth.[39] TPN can be started immediately on recognition of GOO, and continued at home.

TYPES OF ENTERAL STENTS

In general, enteral stents are composed of differing types of metal alloys with different lengths, diameter, and expansile forces following deployment. Only uncovered stents are currently available in the United States. All currently available enteral stents are designed for through-the-scope deployment and require a therapeutic channel endoscope.[1]

The first stent available for palliation of malignant GOO in the United States was the Enteral Wallstent (Boston Scientific, Natick, MA, USA), which is composed of an uncovered Elgiloy (stainless steel). Its successor, the Enteral Wallflex (Boston Scientific), is available as a nitinol (nickel-titanium) alloy; it has a flared proximal end designed for increased flexibility and decreased migration following deployment.[1] Whereas the Wallstent has bare wire ends, the Wallflex has looped wire ends. There is no evidence that either of these wire ends is superior.

Stents available outside the United States include the Choostent, Hanarostent (MI Tech, Seoul, Korea), and Song duodenal stent (Stentech, Seoul, Korea).[1,40,41] The Choostent is made of a flexible expansible metal and is unique in design in that the central portion of the stent is covered in polyurethane, whereas the uncovered flared ends are not. The Hanarostent is available as an uncovered or partially covered self-expanding nitinol stent. The Song stent is similar to the Choostent in that it has a central polyurethane-covered portion with flared ends.[40]

There are many other stents being developed.[26,42–45] One example is a design proposed by Kim and colleagues[46] to prevent migration, which includes using a covered "stent within stent design" the additional application of 3 endoscopic clips to the proximal end helps to anchor the stent in place.

INDICATIONS FOR ENTERAL STENT PLACEMENT

Enteral stents are indicated in patients with confirmed malignant GOO, diagnosed through history, physical examination, imaging, and endoscopy. Enteral stents are frequently employed in patients who are poor surgical candidates with shortened life expectancy, advanced or metastatic disease, significant medical comorbidities, and known anesthesia risk.[1,7,47,48]

Surgery, in comparison with enteral stents, is superior in patients with a longer life expectancy because of lower rates of reobstruction. It is difficult to delineate the survival time preferable for surgery, as it is difficult to predict life expectancy.[12] Adler and Baron[7] have proposed an algorithm for patient selection and treatment options, which has been validated by other studies.[35] The algorithm suggests that if a patient has a resectable malignancy then surgical resection should be attempted. If subsequently found to be unresectable at the time of surgery, but localized, and the patient has a good performance status, then a gastrojejunostomy is probably the best option. If the individual has poor performance status, widespread disease, or a severe medical comorbidity, abdominal CT scan and/or UGI series with small bowel follow-through should be obtained. If there is a single site of obstruction and no evidence of peritoneal carcinomatosis, enteral stent placement is the preferred option. If multiple sites of obstruction and/or peritoneal carcinomatosis are identified, a palliative nasoenteric feeding tube or TPN with gastric decompression would be a suitable option.[7]

CONTRAINDICATIONS

Contraindications to the placement of an enteral stent are relatively few, and include multiple gastrointestinal tract obstructions (often seen in patients with peritoneal carcinomatosis), life expectancy less than 2 weeks, and underlying gastric dysmotility.[7,47,48] Multiple sites of obstruction from metastatic disease and sites that cannot be reached endoscopically (such as the mid to distal jejunum) are contraindications. If life expectancy is less than 1 month, or there are gastric motility problems including linitis plastica, Wai and colleagues[47] have suggested that placement of a nasoenteric tube with gastric decompression is more beneficial.

ENTERAL STENT EFFICACY AND OUTCOMES

Technical success in placing an enteral stent is defined as adequate positioning and deployment of the stent (**Fig. 2**).[17] Technical success ranges anywhere from 75% to 100% in various studies.[21,27,44,46,49–57] One large review article containing data on 1046 patients receiving enteral stents cited technical success in 96%.[17] Common reasons for technical failure include the inability to pass a guide wire across the stricture, inability to advance the stent catheter across the stricture (rare), failure of the delivery system to release the stent, failure of stent deployment, and migration of the stent during the procedure.[17,49]

Clinical success with enteral stent placement is defined as relief of symptoms and/or improvement of oral intake.[17] The GOO scoring system (GOOSS) was created to objectively quantify the patient's level of oral intake both before and following

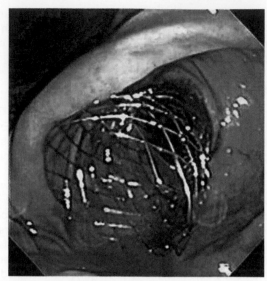

Fig. 2. Endoscopic Image of a well-placed, fully deployed enteral stent bridging the pylorus in a patient with GOO secondary to pancreatic cancer.

treatment.[7] While other scoring systems have b created, the GOOSS is considered the standard scoring system for assessing clinical success in response to treatment of GOO via any method.[17,41] The GOOSS uses a score of 0 for no oral intake, a score of 1 for ability to consume liquids only, a score of 2 for soft solids, and a score of 3 for a low-residue or full diet (**Table 1**).[7,17]

Clinical success rates in recent studies range from 63% to 97%.[7,30,41] Dormann and colleagues[58] analyzed 32 studies with primary data and reported clinical success in 89% of 589 patients following successful stent placement. Patients in this analysis had a mean GOOSS score of 0.4 before stent placement, which increased to a mean of 2.4 following stent placement. The investigators reported that the mean time to overall resolution of symptoms was 4 days, with a range of 1 to 7 days.[58] Reasons for clinical failure occurred in 65 patients, due to disease progression (61%), early stent migration (20%), and procedural-related causes (15%) including the stent being deployed too far proximally or distally, or from inadequate expansion on deployment. In the remaining patients no cause was cited.[58]

Another large review article by Jeurnink and colleagues[17] examined 44 publications with a total of 1000 patients receiving duodenal stents. Clinical success was 89%.

Table 1 The gastric outlet obstruction scoring system	
Score	**Level of Oral Intake**
0	No oral intake
1	Liquids only
2	Soft solids
3	Low-residue or full diet

Data from Adler DG, Baron TH. Endoscopic palliation of malignant gastric outlet obstruction using self-expanding metal stents: experience in 36 patients. Am J Gastroenterol 2002;97(1):72–8.

Before intervention GOOSS scores were 0 in 62%, 1 in 33%, and 2 in 5%. Following stent placement GOOSS scores were 0 in 6%, 1 in 22%, 2 in 40%, and 3 in 32%. Most patients were able to tolerate an oral diet within 24 hours of stent placement.[1,7,30,58]

Hospital stays following enteral stent placement range from 0 (outpatient) to 18 days.[1,59] Average hospital time for 324 patients following enteral stent placement was 7 days.[17] In the United States most enteral stents are placed as an outpatient procedure.

LIFE EXPECTANCY FOLLOWING PLACEMENT OF AN ENTERAL STENT

Enteral stents are generally indicated in patients with unresectable malignancies and symptomatic GOO.[7,35] Multiple studies have shown that mean survival following an enteral stent placement is approximately 12 weeks, which is not surprising given the advanced nature of tumors that cause GOO.[7,17,58] Patients with malignant GOO tend to have similar survival times regardless of the type of cancer involved.[60]

QUALITY OF LIFE

Restoration of the ability to eat, drink, and take medications by mouth is greatly desired by patients with malignant GOO, and almost all patients who have a good clinical outcome following the placement of an enteral stent report satisfaction with the improvement in their situation. Most, but not all, studies have shown an improvement in quality of life following enteral stenting. In a study of 51 patients receiving a Wallflex enteral stent, Van Hooft and colleagues[61] found no significant improvement in the quality of life with scoring systems such as the European Organization for Research and Treatment of Cancer, version 3, and EQ-5D including the EuroQol Visual Analog Scale ($P = .52, .31$, respectively). By comparison, Lowe and colleagues[16] found that Karnofsky scores improved from 44 to 63 following stenting (95% CI 15–22.3, $P<.001$). Mehta and colleagues[20] showed similar improvements in quality of life in 10 patients using the short-form 36 questionnaire at 1 month ($P<.01$). Other studies have shown similar improvements in quality of life.[18,19]

COMPLICATIONS

Complications are frequently categorized into either early ($\leq$7 days), or late (>7 days), and either major or minor.[17] Minor complications, which are non–life threatening, include mild pain, mild fever, and/or occasional vomiting without obstruction. Major complications, defined as severe and life threatening, include but are not limited to perforation, fistula formation, stent migration, hemorrhage, fever, and severe pain.[17] Complication rates range from 0% to 30% depending on the definition of complications used and the inclusion or exclusion of minor complications such as nausea and vomiting.[5,7,20,62]

In a large review, minor complications occurred in 9% of 732 patients. Early major complications occurred in 7% of 609 patients, and were most likely secondary to stent dysfunction, migration, aspiration, bleeding, and perforation.[7,10] Many patients with early major complications, such as stent dysfunction and migration, received a second intervention via endoscopy, including the placement of a second stent. Late major complications occurred in 18% of 950 patients. Late major complications were most commonly stent migration, occlusion either secondary to food or tumor ingrowth/overgrowth, and/or perforation.[10,17] Tumor ingrowth refers to growth of the tumor through the interstices of the stent, and overgrowth refers to growth beyond the length a previously placed stent (**Fig. 3**).[1] Reintervention following obstruction occurred in 18% of patients.[17]

In a recent prospective study of 51 patients, a representative sample of complications was seen. Complications included intermittent pain (8%), cholangitis (6%), bleeding (8%), and migration (2%). Complications such as pain were treated with analgesics, cholangitis with antibiotics and percutaneous drainage, and bleeding with radiotherapy and endoscopic reintervention. The investigators also reported clinical suspicion of stent dysfunction (24%), and endoscopic evidence of tumor overgrowth (10%) and ingrowth (2%). Stent complications secondary to tumor overgrowth and ingrowth were treated with placement of a second stent.[2]

In a review of 606 patients, an overall complication rate of 28% was seen. Major complications included perforation (1.2%), bleeding (0.5%), stent obstruction (17.2%), migration (5.1%), and biliary complications (1.3%). Minor complications included pain (2.5%) and other unspecified complications (0.7%).[58]

In a prospective study of 45 patients, 2 patients developed a duodenal perforation secondary to guide wire and/or biliary stent placement. Both were surgically managed. One stent migration occurred.[41]

Kim and colleagues[32] performed a prospective cohort study of 213 patients. Following enteral stent placement, the overall complication rate was 21%. Major complications included bleeding (1%), tumor overgrowth (7%), stent collapse (4%), food impaction (2%), migration (4%), and jaundice (2%). Minor complications included the formation of granulation tissue (1%). Placement of a second stent and was used to manage stent obstruction. One migration was treated with surgical removal. Food impaction was treated with endoscopic removal.

ROLE OF BILIARY STENTS WITH ENTERAL STENTS

Biliary obstruction can develop concomitantly with GOO or at a later date.[28] Seventy percent to 90% of patients with pancreatic adenocarcinoma will eventually develop biliary obstruction. In one retrospective study of 36 patients with GOO due to a variety

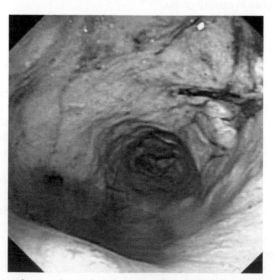

Fig. 3. Tumor In growth seen through the lumen of an enteral stent placed 6 months previously in a patient with metastatic melanoma to the small bowel.

of cancers (6%), 44% of these also had malignant biliary obstruction. Biliary obstruction was observed in 56% prior to GOO, concomitantly in 25%, and following development of GOO in 19%.[7] Drainage of the biliary tree was performed surgically (biliary-enteric bypass) and with biliary stent placement percutaneously, and endoscopically.[63] In 16 patients endoscopic retrograde cholangiopancreatographic placement of a biliary stent was attempted and was successful in 11. Of the 5 remaining patients percutaneous placement of a biliary stent was attempted and was successful in 4. The remaining patient declined further intervention.[7]

Endoscopic approaches to treat biliary obstruction are most commonly employed. Endoscopic placement of a biliary stent is preferred for the alleviation of jaundice and pruritus in comparison with either surgical biliary-enteric bypass or percutaneous trans-hepatic access. This preference for endoscopic placement of biliary stents is secondary to better quality-of-life measurements, decreased length of hospitalization, decreased procedure-related complications and mortality, and decreased overall cost.[63–67]

Simultaneous placement of a biliary stent should be strongly considered when placing an enteral stent for GOO. It has been shown that technical success rates and immediate procedural complications following placement of both a biliary and enteral stent are comparable to placement of an enteral stent alone.[63,68] If there concern for impending or future biliary obstruction, strong consideration should be given to placement of a prophylactic metal biliary stent.

If an enteral stent has already been placed in the duodenum, accessing the papilla can be difficult. If biliary obstruction occurs following placement of an enteral stent and the papilla cannot be accessed, percutaneous and surgical approaches may allow stenting to be completed.[28]

ENTERAL STENTS IN COMPARISON WITH GASTROJEJUNOSTOMY

Many studies have been published that compare indications, enteral stents, and gastrojejunostomy.[12,16–20,35,48,69–71] A retrospective study by Del Piano and colleagues[35] compared 24 patients with enteral stent placement and 23 patients who underwent open gastrojejunostomy for unresectable malignancies. Technical success rates were similar, but the stent group had a higher clinical success rate (92% vs 56%, $P = .0067$), shorter hospital stays (1.4 vs 10.3, $P<.001$), reduced 30-day mortality rates (0% vs 30%, $P = .004$), and less associated morbidity (17% vs 61%, $P = .0021$).

A prospective randomized trial (SUSTENT study) conducted by Jeurnink and colleagues[12] compared open and laparoscopic gastrojejunostomy with enteral stent placement. There were 18 patients randomized to gastrojejunostomy and 21 to enteral stents. Food intake improved more rapidly following stent placement than following gastrojejunostomy (5 vs 8 days, $P<.01$), but long-term relief was better with gastrojejunostomy (50 vs 72 days, $P = .05$). However, more recurrent obstructive symptoms (8 vs 1, $P = .02$), and reinterventions (10 vs 2, $P<.01$) were seen in the enteral stents group. There was no significant difference in complication rates when stent obstruction was not included as a complication, and there was no difference in median survival and quality-of-life scores.

When examining different trials of stent placement and gastrojejunostomy no differences are seen in technical success (96% vs 100%), early (7% vs 6%) and late (18% vs 17%) major complications, and persistent symptoms (8% vs 9%). Initial clinical success is higher after stent placement (89% vs 72), with shorter hospital stays (7 vs 13 days) but with a higher rate of reobstruction (18% vs 1%).[17]

These results show that enteral stent placement is likely favorable in patients with a shorter life expectancy and/or who are poor surgical candidates.

STENT PLACEMENT FOLLOWING SURGERY

GOO following surgical gastrectomy due to recurrent disease with or without distant metastases occurs in approximately 20% of patients.[44,72] Surgical anastomotic sites are an independent risk factor for GOO.[52] Many patients with recurrent malignancies are not candidates for repeat surgical procedures, due to the associated morbidity and mortality.[35,44,73–76] Recurrent GOO following surgery is an appropriate indication for placement of an enteral stent.[44,52] One retrospective study of 20 patients with recurrent malignant obstruction showed a lower restenosis rate with the use of a simultaneously placed uncovered and covered stent in comparison with an uncovered stent alone (0 vs 5 patients, $P = .033$).[44] Fluoroscopy and direct visualization had similar technical and clinical success rates in comparison with patients with no prior surgeries.[77]

COST COMPARISONS

Cost differences between enteral stent placement and surgical procedures have been compared in multiple studies.[7,15,17,21,62,78,79] Webb and colleagues retrospectively compared 10 patients who received an enteral stent with 10 patients who underwent open gastrojejunostomy. Procedural and hospitalization costs were found to be $5970 for enteral stents in comparison with $13,445 for surgical bypass ($P<.0001$). Decreased hospital stay was the primary reason for decreased costs of enteral stent placement.[7,78] In a retrospective study, Yim and colleagues[25] reported procedural cost data on 29 patients receiving an enteral stent and 15 patients undergoing open palliative gastrojejunostomy. Mean cost of enteral stent placement was $9921 in comparison with $28,173 for open gastrojejunostomy ($P<.005$). Mittal and colleagues[62] reported procedural and postprocedural costs in 56 patients undergoing open gastrojejunostomy (New Zealand $13,256), with 14 patients undergoing laparoscopic gastrojejunostomy (New Zealand $10,938) and 16 patients undergoing enteral stent placement (New Zealand $5,736) for malignant GOO. Johnsson and colleagues[79] included procedure, postoperative care, hospital stay, and additional procedures in overall cost analysis in a prospective study of 21 patients undergoing enteral stent placement and 15 patients undergoing open gastrojejunostomy. Mean costs were $7215 for enteral stents and $10,190 for open gastrojejunostomy ($P<.05$).

A multicenter study in the Netherlands randomized 21 patients to enteral stent placement and 18 to gastrojejunostomy (16 open gastrojejunostomy, 2 laparoscopic gastrojejunostomy patients). Initial costs were lower for enteral stent placement (€4820 vs €8315, $P<.001$). There was no difference seen in follow-up costs in the two groups. Overall, costs for enteral stents were significantly lower than for enteral stent placement (€8819 vs €12,433, $P = .049$).[15]

All previous studies have shown that enteral stent placement is more cost effective in comparison with gastrojejunostomy, likely due to decreased length of hospital stay and decreased initial workforce requirement at the time of procedure.

SUMMARY

Malignant GOO remains a commonly encountered clinical entity. GOO is most commonly diagnosed through an appropriate history, physical examination, imaging studies, and evidence found during upper endoscopy. Treatment most commonly includes open or laparoscopic surgical gastrojejunostomy, or enteral stent placement.

Other treatment options include radiation, chemotherapy, nasoenteric tube placement, and TPN.

Technical and clinical success rates for enteral stent placement are, in general, extremely high. Complications include mild pain, fever, vomiting, perforation, fistula formation, stent migration, stent obstruction, and hemorrhage and/or severe pain, but major complications are relatively uncommon. Biliary stent placement should be strongly considered concomitantly with enteral stent placement.

Enteral stent placement, in comparison with surgical options, is better suited for patients with a shorter life expectancy and/or those patients who are poor surgical candidates. Gastrojejunostomy is more beneficial in patients with resectable disease and longer life expectancies. Enteral stent placement is a cost-effective procedure for the palliation of GOO.

REFERENCES

1. Frech EJ, Adler DG. Endoscopic therapy for malignant bowel obstruction. J Support Oncol 2007;5(7):303–10, 319.
2. Van Hooft JE, Dijkgraaf MG, Timmer R, et al. Independent predictors of survival in patients with incurable malignant gastric outlet obstruction: a multicenter prospective observational study. Scand J Gastroenterol 2010;45(10):1217–22.
3. SEER Pancreatic Cancer Statistics, National Cancer Institute. Available at: http://seer.cancer.gov/csr/1975_2007/results_merged/sect_22_pancreas.pdf. Accessed October 26, 2010.
4. SEER Gastric Cancer Statistics. National Cancer Institute. Available at: http://seer.cancer.gov/csr/1975_2007/results_merged/sect_24_stomach.pdf. Accessed October 26, 2010.
5. Espinel J, Vivas S, Munoz F, et al. Palliative treatment of malignant obstruction of gastric outlet using an endoscopically placed enteral Wallstent. Dig Dis Sci 2001; 46:2322–4.
6. Lopera JE, Brazzini A, Gonzales A, et al. Gastroduodenal stent placement: current status. Radiographics 2004;24:1561–73.
7. Adler DG, Baron TH. Endoscopic palliation of malignant gastric outlet obstruction using self-expanding metal stents: experience in 36 patients. Am J Gastroenterol 2002;97(1):72–8.
8. Mauro MA, Koehler RE, Baron TH. Advances in gastrointestinal interventions: the treatment of gastroduodenal and colorectal obstructions with metallic stents. Radiology 2000;215:659–69.
9. Kaw M, Singh S, Gagneja H, et al. Role of self expandable metal stents in the palliation of malignant duodenal obstruction. Surg Endosc 2003;17:646–50.
10. Gaidos JK, Draganov PV. Treatment of malignant gastric outlet obstruction with endoscopically placed self-expandable metal stents. World J Gastroenterol 2009;15(35):4365–71.
11. Cho YK, Kim SW, Hur WH, et al. Clinical outcomes of self-expandable metal stent and prognostic factors for stent patency in gastric outlet obstruction caused by gastric cancer. Dig Dis Sci 2010;55(3):668–74.
12. Jeurnink SM, Steyerberg EW, Van Hooft JE, et al. Surgical gastrojejunostomy or endoscopic stent placement for the palliation of malignant gastric outlet obstruction (SUSTENT study): a multicenter randomized trial. Gastrointest Endosc 2010;71(3):490–9.
13. Keranen I, Udd M, Lepisto A, et al. Outcome for self-expandable metal stents in malignant gastroduodenal obstruction: single-center experience with 104 patients. Surg Endosc 2009. [Epub ahead of print].

14. Kim HJ, Park JY, Bang S, et al. Self-expandable metal stents for recurrent malignant obstruction after gastric surgery. Hepatogastroenterology 2009;56(91/92):914–7.
15. Jeurnink SM, Polinder S, Steverberg EW, et al. Cost comparison of gastrojejunos-tomy versus duodenal stent placement for malignant gastric outlet obstruction. J Gastroenterol 2010;45(5):537–43.
16. Lowe AS, Beckett CG, Jowett S, et al. Self-expandable metal stent placement for the palliation of malignant gastroduodenal obstruction: experience in a large, single, UK centre. Clin Radiol 2007;62(8):738–44.
17. Jeurnink SM, van Eijck CH, Steyerberg EW, et al. Stent versus gastrojejunos-tomy for the palliation of gastric outlet obstruction: a systematic review. BMC Gastroenterol 2007;7:18.
18. Stawowy M, Kruse A, Mortensen FV, et al. Endoscopic stenting for malignant gastric outlet obstruction. Surg Laparosc Endosc Percutan Tech 2007;17(1):5–9.
19. Fiocca E, Ceci V, Donatelli G, et al. Palliative treatment of upper gastrointestinal obstruction using self-expansible metal stents. Eur Rev Med Pharmacol Sci 2006;10(4):179–82.
20. Mehta S, Hindmarsh A, Cheong E, et al. Prospective randomized trial of laparo-scopic gastrojejunostomy versus duodenal stenting for malignant gastric outflow obstruction. Surg Endosc 2006;20(2):239–42.
21. Kim JH, Song HY, Shin JH, et al. Metallic stent placement in the palliative treat-ment of malignant gastric outlet obstructions: primary gastric carcinoma versus pancreatic carcinoma. AJR Am J Roentgenol 2009;193(1):241–7.
22. Larseen I, Medhus AW, Hauge T. Treatment of malignant gastric outlet obstruction with stents: an evaluation of the reported variables for clinical outcome. BMC Gastroenterol 2009;9:45.
23. Kiely JM, Dua KS, Graewin SJ, et al. Palliative stenting for late malignant gastric outlet obstruction. J Gastrointest Surg 2007;11(1):107–13.
24. Telford JJ, Carr-Locke DL, Baron TH, et al. Palliation of patients with malignant gastric outlet obstruction with the enteral Wallstent: outcomes from a multicenter study. Gastrointest Endosc 2004;60(6):916–20.
25. Yim HB, Jacobson BC, Saltzman JR, et al. Clinical outcome of the use of enteral stents for palliation of patients with malignant upper GI obstruction. Gastrointest Endosc 2001;53(3):329–32.
26. Song HY, Shin JH, Yoon CJ, et al. A dual expandable nitinol stent: experience in 102 patients with malignant gastroduodenal strictures. J Vasc Interv Radiol 2004; 15(12):1443–9.
27. Lindsay JO, Andreyev HJ, Vlavianos P, et al. Self-expanding metal stents for the palliation of malignant gastroduodenal obstruction in patients unsuitable for surgical bypass. Aliment Pharmacol Ther 2004;19(8):901–5.
28. Adler DG, Merwat SN. Endoscopic approaches for palliation of luminal gastroin-testinal obstruction. Gastroenterol Clin North Am 2006;35(1):65–82, viii.
29. Lau JY, Chung SC, Sung JJ, et al. Through-the-scope balloon dilation for pyloric stenosis: long-term results. Gastrointest Endosc 1996;43(2 Pt 1):98–101.
30. Holt AP, Patel M, Ahmed MM. Palliation of patients with malignant gastroduodenal obstruction with self-expanding metallic stents: the treatment of choice? Gastro-intest Endosc 2004;60(6):1010–7.
31. Im JP, Kang JM, Kim SG, et al. Clinical outcomes and patency of self-expanding metal stents in patients with malignant upper gastrointestinal obstruction. Dig Dis Sci 2008;53(4):938–45.
32. Kim JH, Song HY, Shin JH, et al. Metallic stent placement in the palliative treat-ment of malignant gastroduodenal obstructions: prospective evaluation of results

and factors influencing outcome in 213 patients. Gastrointest Endosc 2007;66(2): 256–64.

33. Wilson RG, Varma JS. Laparoscopic gastroenterostomy for malignant duodenal obstruction. Br J Surg 1992;79:1348.

34. Ly J, O'Grady G, Mittal A, et al. A systematic review of methods to palliate malignant gastric outlet obstruction. Surg Endosc 2010;24(2):290–7.

35. Del Piano M, Ballare M, Montino F, et al. Endoscopy or surgery for malignant GI outlet obstruction? Gastrointest Endosc 2005;61(3):421–6.

36. Mogavero GT, Jones B, Cameron JL, et al. Gastric and duodenal obstruction in patients with cholangiocarcinoma in the porta hepatis: increased prevalence after radiation therapy. AJR Am J Roentgenol 1992;159(5):1001–3.

37. Park JJ, Lee YC, Kim BK, et al. Long-term clinical outcomes of self-expanding metal stents for treatment of malignant gastroesophageal junction obstructions and prognostic factors for stent patency: effects of anticancer treatments. Dig Liver Dis 2010;42(6):436–40.

38. Guedon C. Enteral nutrition: techniques and indications. Ann Med Interne (Paris) 2000;151(8):659–63 [in French].

39. Otabor IA, Abdessalam SF, Erdman SH, et al. Gastric outlet obstruction due to adenocarcinoma in a patient with Ataxia-Telangiectasia syndrome: a case report and review of the literature. World J Surg Oncol 2009;7:29.

40. Chun HJ, Kim ES, Hyun JJ, et al. Gastrointestinal and biliary stents. J Gastroenterol Hepatol 2010;25(2):234–43.

41. Havemann MC, Adamsen S, Wøjdemann M. Malignant gastric outlet obstruction managed by endoscopic stenting: a prospective single-centre study. Scand J Gastroenterol 2009;44(2):248–51.

42. Seo EH, Jung MK, Park MJ, et al. Covered expandable nitinol stents for malignant gastroduodenal obstructions. J Gastroenterol Hepatol 2008;23(7 Pt 1):1056–62.

43. Maetani I, Isayama H, Mizumoto Y. Palliation in patients with malignant gastric outlet obstruction with a newly designed enteral stent: a multicenter study. Gastrointest Endosc 2007;66(2):355–60.

44. Song GA, Kang DH, Kim TO, et al. Endoscopic stenting in patients with recurrent malignant obstruction after gastric surgery: uncovered versus simultaneously deployed uncovered and covered (double) self-expandable metal stents. Gastrointest Endosc 2007;65(6):782–7.

45. Bessoud B, de Baere T, Denys A, et al. Malignant gastroduodenal obstruction: palliation with self-expanding metallic stents. J Vasc Interv Radiol 2005;16(2 Pt 1): 247–53.

46. Kim ID, Kang DH, Choi CW, et al. Prevention of covered enteral stent migration in patients with malignant gastric outlet obstruction: a pilot study of anchoring with endoscopic clips. Scand J Gastroenterol 2010;45(1):100–5.

47. Wai CT, Ho KY, Yeoh KG, et al. Palliation of malignant gastric outlet obstruction caused by gastric cancer with self-expandable metal stents. Surg Laparosc Endosc Percutan Tech 2001;11(3):161–4.

48. Kazi HA, O'Reilly DA, Satchidanand RY, et al. Endoscopic stent insertion for the palliation of malignant gastric outlet obstruction. Dig Surg 2006;23(1/2):28–31.

49. Park KB, Do YS, Kang WK, et al. Malignant obstruction of gastric outlet and duodenum: palliation with flexible covered metallic stents. Radiology 2001;219(3): 679–83.

50. Huang Q, Dai DK, Qian XJ, et al. Treatment of gastric outlet and duodenal obstructions with uncovered expandable metal stents. World J Gastroenterol 2007;13(40): 5376–9.

51. Kim TO, Kang DH, Kim GH, et al. Self-expandable metallic stents for palliation of patients with malignant gastric outlet obstruction caused by stomach cancer. World J Gastroenterol 2007;13(6):916–20.

52. Kim GH, Kang DH, Lee DH, et al. Which types of stent, uncovered or covered, should be used in gastric outlet obstructions? Scand J Gastroenterol 2004; 39(10):1010–4.

53. Schiefke I, Zabel-Langhennig A, Wiedmann M, et al. Self-expandable metallic stents for malignant duodenal obstruction caused by biliary tract cancer. Gastrointest Endosc 2003;58(2):213–9.

54. Johnston SD, McKelvey ST, Moorehead RJ, et al. Duodenal stents for malignant duodenal strictures. Ulster Med J 2002;71(1):30–3.

55. Jeong JY, Han JK, Kim AY, et al. Fluoroscopically guided placement of a covered self-expandable metallic stent for malignant antroduodenal obstructions: preliminary results in 18 patients. AJR Am J Roentgenol 2002;178(4):847–52.

56. Pinto IT. Malignant gastric and duodenal stenosis: palliation by peroral implantation of a self-expanding metallic stent. Cardiovasc Intervent Radiol 1997;20(6): 431–4.

57. Profili S, Meloni GB, Bifulco V, et al. Self-expandable metal stents in the treatment of antro-pyloric and/or duodenal strictures. Acta Radiol 2001;42(2):176–80.

58. Dormann A, Meisner S, Verin N, et al. Self-expanding metal stents for gastroduodenal malignancies: systematic review of their clinical effectiveness. Endoscopy 2004;36(6):543–50.

59. Kim JH, Yoo BM, Lee KJ, et al. Self-expanding coil stent with a long delivery system for palliation of unresectable malignant gastric outlet obstruction: a prospective study. Endoscopy 2001;33(10):838–42.

60. Shaw JM, Bornman PC, Krige JE, et al. Self-expanding metal stents as an alternative to surgical bypass for malignant gastric outlet obstruction. Br J Surg 2010; 97(6):872–6.

61. van Hooft JE, Uitdehaag MJ, Bruno MJ, et al. Efficacy and safety of the new WallFlex enteral stent in palliative treatment of malignant gastric outlet obstruction (DUO-FLEX study): a prospective multicenter study. Gastrointest Endosc 2009;69(6): 1059–66.

62. Mittal A, Windsor J, Woodfield J, et al. Matched study of three methods for palliation of malignant pyloroduodenal obstruction. Br J Surg 2004;28:812–7.

63. Srikureja W, Chang KJ. Endoscopic palliation of pancreatic adenocarcinoma. Curr Opin Gastroenterol 2005;21(5):601–5.

64. Smith AC, Dowsett JF, Russell RC, et al. Randomised trial of endoscopic stenting versus surgical bypass in malignant low bile duct obstruction. Lancet 1994;344: 1655–60.

65. Speer AG, Cotton PB, Russell RC, et al. Randomised trial of endoscopic versus percutaneous stent insertion in malignant obstructive jaundice. Lancet 1987;2: 57–62.

66. Brandabur JJ, Kozarek RA, Ball TJ, et al. Nonoperative versus operative treatment of obstructive jaundice in pancreatic cancer: cost and survival analysis. Am J Gastroenterol 1988;83:1132–9.

67. Shepherd HA, Royle G, Ross AP, et al. Endoscopic biliary endoprosthesis in the palliation of malignant obstruction of the distal common bile duct: a randomized trial. Br J Surg 1988;75:1166–8.

68. Kaw M, Singh S, Gagneja H. Clinical outcome of simultaneous self-expandable metal stents for palliation of malignant biliary and duodenal obstruction. Surg Endosc 2003;17:457–61.

69. Artifon EL, Sakai P, Cunha JE, et al. Surgery or endoscopy for palliation of biliary obstruction due to metastatic pancreatic cancer. Am J Gastroenterol 2006; 101(9):2031–7.
70. Espinel J, Sanz O, Vivas S, et al. Malignant gastrointestinal obstruction: endoscopic stenting versus surgical palliation. Surg Endosc 2006;20(7):1083–7.
71. Sunpaweravong S, Ovartlarnporn B, Khow-ean U, et al. Endoscopic stenting versus surgical bypass in advanced malignant distal bile duct obstruction: cost effectiveness analysis. Asian J Surg 2005;28(4):262–5.
72. Iwanaga T, Koyama H, Furukawa H, et al. Mechanisms of late recurrence after radical surgery for gastric carcinoma. Am J Surg 1978;135:637–40.
73. Monson JR, Donohue JH, Mcllrath DC, et al. Total gastrectomy for advanced cancer: a worthwhile palliative procedure. Cancer 1991;68:1863–8.
74. Morgoshiia TSh, Guliaev AV. Assessment of the intermediate and the late results of surgery for gastric stump cancer. Vopr Onkol 2003;49:752–4 [in Russian].
75. Weaver DW, Wiencek RG, Bouwman DL, et al. Gastrojejunostomy: is it helpful for patients with pancreatic cancer? Surgery 1987;102:608–13.
76. Baines MJ. Management of intestinal obstruction in patients with advanced cancer. Ann Acad Med Singapore 1994;23:178–82.
77. Lee JM, Han YM, Kim CS, et al. Fluoroscopic-guided covered metallic stent placement for gastric outlet obstruction and post-operative gastroenterostomy anastomotic stricture. Clin Radiol 2001;56(7):560–7.
78. Webb BM, Baron TH. Endoscopic versus surgical palliation of malignant gastric outlet obstruction: a retrospective analysis [abstract]. Gastrointest Endosc 2000; 51:AB221.
79. Johnsson E, Thune A, Liedman B. Palliation of malignant gastroduodenal obstruction with open surgical bypass or endoscopic stenting: clinical outcome and health economic evaluation. World J Surg 2004;28:812–7.

Plastic Biliary Stents for Benign Biliary Diseases

Vincenzo Perri, MD, Pietro Familiari, MD, PhD,
Andrea Tringali, MD, PhD, Ivo Boskoski, MD,
Guido Costamagna, MD*

KEYWORDS

- Benign biliary diseases • Biliary strictures • Plastic biliary stents
- Stent therapy

Plastic stents were the first endoprostheses used for the management of biliary disease. The first biliary stent placement was reported in the late seventies by Soehendra and Reynders-Frederix,[1] for the palliation of a malignant biliary stricture.

Since then, biliary plastic stent placement has become a well-established technique for numerous indications. The procedure already has a universally recognized role in the management of malignant biliary obstruction, and biliary plastic stents are now gaining consensus for the treatment of a variety of benign biliary disorders. The spectrum of benign diseases amenable to endoscopic stenting has expanded in recent years and currently includes postoperative biliary injuries, including leaks and strictures, dominant biliary strictures in primary sclerosing cholangitis, chronic pancreatitis, cholecystitis, and large nonremovable biliary stones.

The outcomes of plastic stent placement for the management of benign biliary disorders are summarized in this review. Patient selection and indications for stent placement are discussed, and some technical hints for stent placement in the various clinical scenarios are provided.

POSTOPERATIVE BILIARY INJURIES
Bile Duct Leak

Bile leaks are most often a consequence of surgery (open and laparoscopic cholecystectomy, liver transplantation, and major hepatic surgery) or trauma. Endoscopic treatment aims at reducing the pressure gradient between the biliary tree and the duodenum to promote preferential bile flow into the duodenum and allow the leak to seal.[2] This outcome can be accomplished by biliary stenting, biliary sphincterotomy, nasobiliary drainage (NBD), or a combination of these techniques.[3–5] These methods

Digestive Endoscopy Unit, Gemelli University Hospital, Universita' Cattolica del Sacro Cuore, Largo Gemelli 8, Roma 00168, Italy
* Corresponding author.
E-mail address: gcostamagna@rm.unicatt.it

Gastrointest Endoscopy Clin N Am 21 (2011) 405–433
doi:10.1016/j.giec.2011.04.012
1052-5157/11/$ – see front matter © 2011 Elsevier Inc. All rights reserved.

giendo.theclinics.com

seem to be equally effective in facilitating closure of a biliary leak within a few days,[2,6] and the endoscopic approach of choice remains controversial because each option has its own limitations and advantages.

Endoscopic sphincterotomy is associated with immediate, short-term, and long-term complications, but is necessary when dealing with associated residual common bile duct (CBD) stones.

Disadvantages in using NBD include prolonged hospitalization stays while awaiting leak closure, patient discomfort, and tube migration or inadvertent dislodgement. Its main advantage is maintenance of access for repeat cholangiography to confirm leak closure.

Stent placement requires at least 1 repeated procedure for stent removal, more if stent occlusion or migration occurs, but it avoids the need for sphincterotomy. Stents are necessary when a biliary stricture is located distal to a leak.

In an animal study, more rapid closure of a postcholecystectomy cystic duct leak was achieved with stent placement compared with biliary sphincterotomy alone.[7] Endoscopic stent placement seems to be the preferred method of treatment of bile leaks at many centers.[2,8–10] Although some advocate placement of a stent of sufficient length to traverse the site of the bile duct defect,[9] traversing the papilla is often all that is necessary to optimize the pressure gradient for internalization of bile flow.

Nearly all postoperative biliary leaks, with the exception of complete transection of the CBD, which is an indication for reconstructive surgery, are amenable to endoscopic therapy. As early as 1991, Binmoeller and colleagues[6] reported successful healing of biliary leaks in 82% of 77 patients treated endoscopically. These results have been confirmed and improved upon in more recent studies with a greater than 90% success rate in leak closure.[11–15]

Sandha and colleagues[12] proposed the use of biliary sphincterotomy alone to treat small leaks (visualized only after filling of the intrahepatic ducts) and temporary (4–6 weeks) biliary stenting for large leaks (visualized before intrahepatic duct opacification) or in the setting of associated strictures, contraindications to sphincterotomy or inadequate drainage of contrast medium after sphincterotomy. This approach led to leak closure in more than 90% of 207 consecutive patients.

Different stent strategies to manage biliary leaks (stenting with or without sphincterotomy, various stent sizes and stent duration) were proposed and compared, all with similar results. Mavrogiannis and colleagues[13] compared 6 to 8 weeks of stent placement using either a 7 French stent without biliary sphincterotomy or a 10 French stent with biliary sphincterotomy, whereas other investigators[14] compared 4-week stenting using either a 10 or 7 French stent (after biliary sphincterotomy).

Biliary stents have also been successfully used to reestablish the continuity of disrupted sectorial/segmental branches at the level of the main hepatic confluence[16] and for leaks from aberrant bile ducts.[17]

The use of large bore stents (>10 French) is preferred to avoid early clogging and to improve bile flow; stents are usually removed 4 to 8 weeks after insertion.[10]

Postoperative Benign Biliary Strictures

Postoperative benign biliary strictures (POBS) occur most commonly after cholecystectomy and are often the result of direct surgical trauma related to partial or complete transection of the bile duct by clipping or ligation. Another mechanism for POBS development is an ischemic insult of the biliary wall caused by dissection or thermal injury.

POBS are usually diagnosed within 6 to 12 months from surgery, and patients may present with jaundice, recurrent cholangitis, abdominal pain, pruritus, bile duct stone formation, and even secondary biliary cirrhosis. Liver biochemistries usually show anicteric cholestasis. Careful evaluation by noninvasive imaging techniques (mainly magnetic resonance cholangio pancreatography [MRCP]) is advisable to plan the treatment strategy.

Bismuth and Lazorthes[18] classified such benign strictures into 5 types:

- Type 1: common bile duct strictures located greater than or equal to 2 cm from the main hepatic confluence
- Type 2: common hepatic duct stricture located less than 2 cm from the main hepatic confluence
- Type 3: ceiling of the biliary confluence is intact, right and left ductal systems communicate
- Type 4: ceiling of the confluence is destroyed, bile ducts are separated
- Type 5: stricture of an isolated aberrant right duct.

When the stricture is close to the hilar confluence, endoscopic management becomes more challenging and needs to be adapted on a case-by-case basis according to the bile duct anatomy.

In a large series, surgical repair of POBS carried a mortality risk close to 2% and relevant morbidity up to 40%.[19,20] Stricture of the bilio-digestive anastomosis is reported in 10% to 15% of cases after 4 to 10 years of follow-up,[20–22] requiring reintervention or repeated percutaneous treatment for prolonged periods of time leading to an impaired quality of life.

Endoscopic treatment of POBS is preferred over percutaneous techniques because it avoids the risk of liver puncture and more easily accesses nondilated intrahepatic ducts. Also, the endoscopic approach is more comfortable for patients because it avoids the need for external drainage.

In the absence of complete transection or ligation of the bile duct, all patients with POBS are candidates for endoscopic treatment. Surgery can be undertaken in cases of failed endotherapy, whereas hepaticojejunostomy makes future endotherapy difficult, if not impossible.

Bergman and colleagues[23] reported on the results of endoscopic stent therapy of POBS in 74 patients using the following protocol: insertion of two 10 French stents whenever possible, planned stent exchange every 3 months, and stent removal at 1 year (so-called Amsterdam protocol). However, because of a variety of reasons, only 59% (44 patients) of the original cohort completed the protocol. The patients were followed for a median time of 9.1 years. Strictures recurred in 20% of patients with the majority presenting within 6 months of stent removal (median 2.6 months, range 2 months to 15 years), potentially because of incomplete treatment. Major complications, including cholangitis, pancreatitis, bleeding, and stent migration, were more common in patients who were noncompliant with the stent exchange protocol.

A more aggressive approach was reported by the authors' institution.[24] At each exchange scheduled every 3 months, all previously placed stents were removed and the maximum number of large-diameter stents inserted, as permitted by the diameter of the duct distal to the stricture and the tightness of the stricture itself. The treatment protocol was stopped when complete morphologic disappearance of the stricture was demonstrated by occlusion cholangiography after stent removal. Complete disappearance of the stricture was defined as absence of any significant indentation at the site of previous narrowing. Of 45 patients, 42 completed the protocol. When compared with the Amsterdam protocol, there was no increase in early and delayed complication rates. Complete morphologic disappearance of the stricture was obtained in 40 patients (89%), with a mean number of 3.2 ± 1.3 stents (range: 1–6) for a mean treatment duration of 12.1 ± 5.3 months (range: 2–24 months).

Two patients died of unrelated causes. The remaining patients were followed for a mean of 4 years without evidence of stricture recurrence and there was 1 case (2.5%) of cholangitis caused by biliary sludge, retreated endoscopically.

These promising results were recently confirmed in the same cohort[25] after a long follow-up (mean 13.7 years, range 11.7–19.8) with a 11.4% stricture recurrence rate, all successfully retreated endoscopically.

Satisfactory results have also been reproduced in a prospective trial involving 43 patients with postlaparoscopic cholecystectomy bile duct strictures in whom a similar aggressive protocol for endoscopic stenting was followed.[26] A mean of 3.4 ± 0.6 (range 3–5) stents were placed for a period of 1 year. The investigators reported a 100% success rate for stricture dilatation with no stricture recurrence at a mean follow up of 16.0 ± 11.1 (range 1–42) months after stent removal.

The major drawback of placement of multiple plastic stents for POBS is the need for repeat endoscopic retrograde cholangiopancreatographies (ERCPs), frequent stent exchanges, and the risk of cholangitis caused by stent dislodgement or poor patient compliance with scheduled stent exchanges.

Endoscopic treatment of POBS needs to be carefully explained to patients and undertaken in those who are willing to accept the 3-monthly stent-exchange schedule. A recall system, especially for patients who are noncompliant, is necessary to prevent cholangitis.

The following are key points and tips for placement of multiple plastic stents in POBS:

1. Use of magnetic resonance cholangiography (MRC) as a roadmap for planning treatment
2. Biliary sphincterotomy to facilitate placement of multiple plastic stents
3. Balloon dilation of strictures to 6 to 8 mm diameter depending on the size of the bile ducts above the stricture
4. Measurement of the distance between the stricture and the papilla using a catheter with radiopaque markers to select the proper stent length
5. Placement of the maximum number of stents (possibly 10 French) in relation to the severity of the stricture and diameter of the bile duct proximal and distal to the stricture
6. Use of angled hydrophilic guidewires to negotiate strictures and pass into intrahepatic ducts to position the catheter where the proximal end of the stent will reside
7. Exchange to stiff guidewires
8. Use of preshaped Cremer hilar stents or a 12-cm long Cotton-Huibregtse (duodenal bend) stent (Cook Endoscopy, Winston Salem, NC, USA) placed upside down (especially when placed into the left hepatic duct) (**Fig. 1**)
9. Stent exchange every 3 months to minimize the risk of stent occlusion-related cholangitis
10. Avoidance of balloon dilation (unless necessary) of the stricture during stent exchanges to reduce trauma to the bile duct
11. Increase the number or the diameter of stents at each stent exchange
12. Treatment duration (stents in place) for at least 12 months
13. Stent removal after complete disappearance of the stricture as visualized by balloon occlusion cholangiography
14. Close clinical and laboratory follow-up (liver function tests obtained every 3 months for the first years then every 6 months) after stent removal to allow for early detection of stricture recurrence.

Endoscopic management of POBS is considered the first-line treatment for most instances. An aggressive approach placing multiple stents improves results and

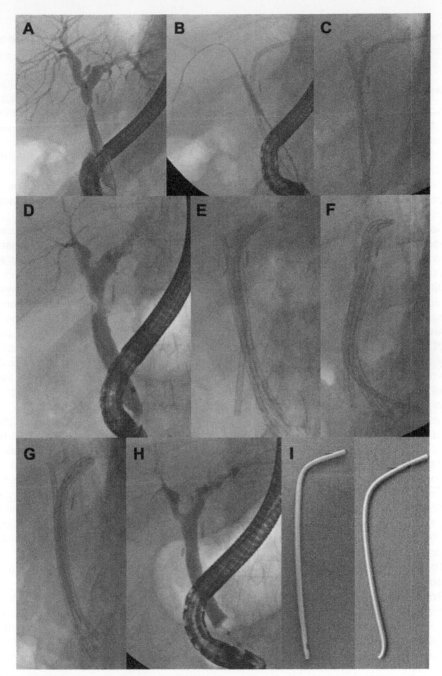

Fig. 1. Multiple stent placements for CBD stricture after cholecystectomy. (*A*) Bismuth type II (<2 cm from the hilar confluence) postoperative bile duct stricture following laparoscopic cholecystectomy, (*B*) balloon dilation, and (*C*) insertion of 2 plastic stents. (*D*) Three months later, stricture improved and (*E*) 5 stents (10 F diameter) were inserted. (*F*) At planned reevaluation, 3 stents had migrated distal to the stricture; (*G*) 5 stents were reinserted (4 in an upside-down position in the left hepatic duct); and (*H*) stents were in place 3 months later, and the stricture completely resolved. (*I*) A Cotton-Huibregtse 12-cm-long stent in upside-down position (*left*) and Cremer hilar stent (*right*).

is the strategy of choice. Surgical reconstruction should be considered for complete transection of the bile duct when endotherapy fails or to treat recurrent strictures.

Biliary Strictures After Liver Transplantation

Endoscopic plastic stent placement is now considered the first-line therapy for biliary strictures that occur after orthotopic liver transplantation (OLT) and living-donor liver transplantation (LDLT).

Biliary strictures occurring after OLT were traditionally managed by surgical repair or balloon dilation, with or without stent insertion, by means of the percutaneous transhepatic route.[27–29] As data accrued on successful management of POBS, ERCP and endoscopic biliary plastic stent placement became the primary therapeutic approach for anastomotic strictures after liver transplantation.[30–36]

Despite the improvements in surgical technique, organ selection, procurement, and preservation, complications of the biliary tract after liver transplantation remain frequent. Strictures account for about 40% of these complications[31] and occur in about 5% to 15% of deceased-donor OLT and 30% of right-lobe LDLT.[31,33,35–54]

Biliary strictures after OLT are classified into 2 main types: anastomotic and nonanastomotic. The incidence, etiology and pathogenesis, presentation, natural history, prognosis, and response to therapy with stent placement differ between the 2 types.

Anastomotic strictures may occur with any biliary anastomosis, whether duct-to-duct or hepaticojejunostomy, in deceased- or living-donor OLT. They are usually solitary strictures and respond favorably to dilation. Anastomotic strictures are the result of improper surgical techniques (excessive use of electrocoagulation, tension at the level of the anastomosis, inappropriate bile duct dissection), small-caliber bile ducts, localized ischemia, infections, or fibrotic healing.[31,34–36]

Nonanastomotic strictures (NAS) may occur anywhere in the biliary tree, either at the level of the hilum, the extrahepatic, or the intrahepatic ducts. They account for 10% to 25% of strictures after OLT. NAS are often multiple, longer than anastomotic strictures, and occur earlier in the postoperative period. Biliary sludge and casts are often associated with nonanastomotic strictures, which are notably difficult to treat and poorly responsive to dilation and nonoperative treatments. Multiple factors contribute to the occurrence of NAS, including ischemia-related injuries, ABO incompatibility, hepatic artery thrombosis (in up to 50% of cases), and immunologic injury to the biliary epithelium.[31,36,55–59] A prolonged cold ischemia time in cadaver donor OLT was significantly associated with the occurrence of NAS.[60,61]

Therefore, differentiation of anastomotic and nonanastomotic strictures is clinically important.

Some prerequisites fundamental and necessary for successful endoscopic plastic stent placement after OLT include duct-to-duct biliary reconstruction and accessibility of the papilla of Vater. Despite case series, endoscopic treatment of biliary strictures in patients with Roux-en-Y hepaticojejunostomy is difficult and challenging. Either a colonoscope or balloon enteroscope is needed to reach the anastomotic site.[62,63]

Although the technique of endoscopic plastic stent placement is well defined and now standardized, there is variability in the treatment of post-OLT biliary strictures based upon review of published studies. Differences include the diameter of stents, diameter of dilating balloons used, the number of side-to-side stents placed, the number of balloon dilations or stent exchanges performed, the time interval between stent exchange, and the overall duration of stent placement. These differences are likely responsible for the large variation in observed outcomes.[64]

Anastomotic strictures

Balloon dilation of anastomotic biliary strictures without stent placement is successful in less than 50% of cases.[65–67]

In a retrospective study of 25 patients with biliary anastomotic strictures, it was found that despite similar immediate success rates, clinically relevant stricture recurrences are more frequent in patients treated with balloon dilation only (recurrence 62%) than in those treated with dilation and stent placement (recurrence 27%).[67] Other investigators have found that a one-time stricture dilation session was effective in only 31.0% of patients, whereas 34.4% of patients required more than 1 balloon dilation session and another one-third required subsequent stent placement.[66] Schwartz and colleagues[65] used small-caliber balloons (4–6 mm) and found balloon dilation alone to be effective in 47% of patients. In a randomized trial that compared balloon dilation alone with balloon dilation and stent placement, dilation alone was as effective as stent placement (sustained clinical success 71% vs 73%).[68] The study was performed on a limited number of patients (n = 32), which included 6 patients with nonanastomotic strictures and 3 with hilar strictures (who had the worst long-term prognosis). Furthermore, in the stent group, patients were usually treated only with the simultaneous placement of few stents (starting with 1 stent, and increasing to a maximum of 3 stents), which may have affected the long-term success rate in the stent group.

Some patients may only have a transient narrowing of a duct-to-duct anastomosis within the first 30 to 60 days after OLT caused by acute edema and inflammation. These strictures respond well to a single session of balloon dilation or placement of a single stent.[34] However, in the vast majority of post-OLT anastomotic strictures, a large-caliber (>6 mm) balloon dilation followed by placement of multiple stents placed side to side appears to be more successful with a durable outcome and is the current preferred approach for the management of anastomotic strictures.[25,31,64,69]

Stent placement for anastomotic strictures is easy when the liver has been transplanted from a deceased donor because the biliary anastomosis is usually located at the level of the middle common bile duct, far from the main biliary confluence.

The technique of placement of multiple plastic stents has been previously described (see POBS section). A distinction of post-OLT biliary strictures, also seen in tight strictures, is that the transplanted liver bile ducts do not display the same degree of proportional dilation as nontransplanted livers. This peculiar behavior has not been completely clarified; however, the presence of fibrosis leading to less pliable ducts has been suggested as a possible etiology.[70] Nevertheless, the absence of substantial dilation of the bile ducts may limit the number of stents that can be placed side to side for the initial stricture dilation.

Large bore stents, 10 or 11.5 French polyethylene stents, are preferred. Standard Cotton-Leung stents (Amsterdam type, central bend) or Cotton-Huibregtse (Cook Endoscopy, Winston Salem, NC, USA) (duodenal bend) stents are chosen for the management of post-OLT anastomotic biliary strictures; they are inexpensive, widely available, available in different calibers and lengths, can be easily tailored or shaped if necessary, and remain patent for a mean of 3 to 4 months. There are isolated reports on the use of inside stents (modified polyethylene endoprostheses that have been placed completely inside the bile ducts, above the papilla of Vater, in an attempt to prolong patency and to reduce the risk of ascending cholangitis). The benefits of such stents have not been demonstrated in controlled trials.[52,53]

The majority of patients with anastomotic biliary strictures that occur after deceased-donor transplantation require several endoscopic interventions (on average between 1.6 and 6.0), with successful long-term clinical and morphologic resolution of the stricture between 70% and 100%. Recurrences have been variably reported in approximately 0% to 20% of cases, but can usually be managed conservatively by repeat endoscopic stent placment.[33,40,41,67–69,71–77] The major disadvantages of endoscopic dilation of anastomotic strictures with plastic stents include the need for multiple procedures repeated over an extended period of time and the risk of cholangitis resulting from stent occlusion. A protocol of accelerated dilation, with plastic stent exchange every 2 weeks and an overall shortened stent period of an average of 3.6 months, showed an 87% success rate.[78]

Patients with anastomotic strictures after OLT require long-term surveillance because strictures may recur, even years after stent removal. Long-term surveillance by liver function test monitoring and noninvasive imaging is advisable. Some investigators have observed that anastomotic strictures that are diagnosed within 6 months after OLT have a better prognosis and response to endoscopic therapy.[31]

Nonanastomotic strictures

In contrast to anastomotic strictures, the management of nonanastomotic strictures after OLT should be individualized. Because of their complex etiology and pathogenesis, nonanastomotic strictures respond less predictably to endoscopic stent placement. Sludge, debris, and casts are commonly found in these patients and may cause early stent occlusion and recurrent cholangitis.[31,34–36,57,58,79]

Stent placement for nonanastomotic strictures is technically demanding and cumbersome. These strictures are usually multiple and variably extend from the proximal common bile duct to the main biliary confluence and sometimes into the intrahepatic branches (**Fig. 2**).

In cases of early hepatic artery thrombosis, emergency revascularization or retransplantation is recommended. For late hepatic artery thrombosis or nonanastomotic strictures unrelated to hepatic artery thrombosis, an attempt at nonoperative management by endoscopic dilation and stent placement is a reasonable approach.

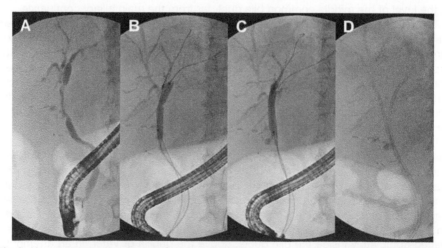

Fig. 2. Nonanastomotic stricture after OLT. Plastic stent placement. (*A*) ERCP showing a nonanastomotic stricture developed 3 months after OLT. The stricture involves the donor common bile duct up to the hilum and the main biliary confluence. (*B, C*) Placement of 2 guidewires, 1 each in the left and right hepatic duct. Balloon dilation of the donor CBD left and right hepatic ducts. (*D*) Placement of 2 plastic biliary stents, 1 each in the left and right hepatic duct (size 8.5 French).

Endoscopic treatment of NAS is similar to that of anastomotic strictures and includes balloon dilation and placement of multiple stents, with the aim of draining all obstructed ducts. There is broad variability in management, but typically smaller-caliber (4–6 mm) balloons and a fewer number of plastic stents are used for NAS strictures because of the small size ducts upstream to the stricture.[32,33] In addition, it is often necessary to use smaller-caliber stents (7–8.5 French).

Some investigators have found that strictures that appear within the first 3 months after OLT were more likely to respond to balloon dilation and stent placement than those with a later presentation.[80]

The mean number of endoscopic procedures needed to achieve satisfactory dilation for nonanastomotic strictures are greater than for anastomotic strictures.[33,81] The outcomes of endoscopic therapy of 12 patients with nonanastomotic strictures were compared with those of 10 patients having anastomotic strictures. Nonanastomotic strictures required significantly longer duration therapy than anastomotic strictures (median 185 vs 67 days, $P = .02$) for successful resolution. Twenty-two months after the first endoscopic treatment, 73% of the donor hepatic-duct-stricture (NAS) group was stent free compared with 90% of the anastomotic group ($P = .02$). Patients with NAS had significantly more hepatic artery thrombosis (58.3% vs 10.0%, $P<.05$), cholangitis (58.3% vs 30.0%), choledocholithiasis (91% vs 10%), and number of endoscopic interventions.[81]

Few studies have directly reported on the outcomes of endoscopic stenting in non-anastomotic strictures. A small number of patients were enrolled in these studies, and the heterogeneous results are difficult to compare. It is common for the response to dilation to be incomplete; morphologic disappearance of the stricture is variable and patients often have persistent cholestasis.[33,58] In addition, long-term antibiotic treatment is required in many patients to treat recurrent cholangitis and intrahepatic abscesses.[35,36,58] Only 50% to 75% of patients with nonanastomotic strictures have a sustained response to stricture dilation and stent placement.[33,58,68,75,76,79,81] Positive outcomes after endoscopic multiple stent placement have been reported by Tabibian and colleagues[79] for 15 patients with nonanastomotic strictures. Nine of the 15 patients had cholangiographic improvement, biochemical normalization, and cholestatic symptom relief; 2 required retransplantation; 1 died of nonbiliary causes; and 3 were still undergoing treatment with stents in place. During a mean follow-up of 17 months, no recurrent strictures were observed in the 9 patients in whom stricture resolution was achieved. In the series reported by Graziadei and colleagues,[33] 19 patients with nonanastomotic strictures underwent stent placement and balloon dilation. After a mean of 8.1 ERCPs, none of the patients achieved complete stricture resolution. All patients had persistent intrahepatic biliary strictures on cholangiogram, whereas 4 patients (21.1%) had complete resolution of clinical symptoms, normal cholestatic parameters, and no significant bile flow impairment. Eight patients (42.1%) also had complete resolution of clinical symptoms but continued to have elevated cholestatic enzymes and significant biliary strictures on cholangiography. No response was seen in 7 patients (36.8%); 4 of these 7 patients required retransplantation (21%) and 3 died (15.8%) of biliary sepsis.

Surgical revision of the biliary anastomosis might be necessary in selected cases after failure of nonoperative management. Early reports suggested that despite attempts at nonoperative management, 25% to 30% of patients with NAS die or undergo retransplantation.[29,33–36,58] Diffuse and extended disease in the smaller intrahepatic ducts is a reason to consider early retransplantation rather than repeated attempts at endoscopic dilation.[35,58] The ischemic events associated with nonanastomotic strictures are responsible for poor graft survival, whereas the overall survival of patients with nonanastomotic strictures is not substantially different from the overall survival of all patients receiving OLT.[33,58] Because of the scarce availability of organs for retransplantation and the lack of effective alternative treatments, endoscopic stent placement may be used as a bridge to retransplantation and occasionally as a palliative option.

Biliary strictures in living-donor liver transplantation

The continuous shortage of deceased-donor organs has urged the transplant community to look for alternative ways of expanding the pool of liver grafts. Over the last 2 decades, living donor liver transplantation has gained acceptance and become a routine alternative in transplant centers. The most frequently used graft in adults is the right liver, using segments V, VI, VII, and VIII. Initially, a Roux-en-Y bilio-jejunal anastomosis was preferred for reconstruction. However, a duct-to-duct biliary anastomosis is being increasingly used, and becoming the favored approach to allow for endoscopic interventions in case of postoperative biliary complications.[31,34]

Biliary strictures are more common in LDLT patients compared with deceased-donor patients, occurring in up to 9% to 43 % of cases.[43,82,83] For duct-to-duct biliary anastomotic strictures, ERCP with endoscopic balloon dilation and plastic stent placement remains the fist-line therapy. Nevertheless, few articles have directly analyzed the role of endoscopy in the management of complications of LDLT and especially treatment of strictures.

The incidence of anastomotic strictures appears to be higher following LDLT than nonanastomotic strictures as compared with recipients of whole-liver grafts.[53,84] Nonanastomotic strictures are probably less frequent because of the short ischemia times and healthy donors.

Patients with duct-to-duct anastomoses LDLT are often complex because there are sometimes multiple anastomoses involving small peripheral ducts, with a high risk of devascularization.[85] Endoscopic plastic stent placement in these patients may be extremely difficult because the location of the anastomosis is variable and often difficult to identify fluoroscopically.

Endoscopic treatment is successful in approximately 60% to 75% of patients with anastomotic biliary strictures after LDLT. Similar to endoscopic treatment of anastomotic strictures in deceased-donor OLT, a combination of balloon dilation and stent placement has been used.[38,41,43,49–54,85–87]

Because of the uncertain outcomes of endoscopic stenting in patients with anastomotic strictures after LDLT, surgical revision of the anastomosis is more frequently performed for LDLT versus deceased-donor OLT.[50]

BILIARY STRICTURES SECONDARY TO CHRONIC PANCREATITIS

Endoscopic plastic stent placement has been widely used for the management of common bile duct strictures in patients with chronic pancreatitis (CP).

CP is an inflammatory process characterized by destruction of pancreatic parenchyma and ductal structures with subsequent formation of fibrosis.[88] CBD strictures can be found in 3% to 46% of patients with advanced CP.[89–96] The true incidence of CP-related CBD strictures is unknown because not all patients present with jaundice, which can be transient.[97]

The nature of the stricture depends on the anatomic relationship of the CBD within the head of the pancreas. Fibrotic CBD strictures occur as a consequence of recurrent acute inflammation in the pancreas, which may eventually result in permanent periductal fibrotic invasion.[98] CBD strictures can also be the result of a focal acute inflammatory process within the pancreatic head or secondary to extrinsic compression from a pancreatic pseudocyst.[99] In these two conditions, the biliary stricture usually resolves after healing of the acute inflammatory process or draining of the pseudocyst, respectively.

The clinical presentation varies from incidentally discovered asymptomatic cholestasis to symptomatic jaundice or cholangitis. The clinical course of the disease is variable and usually characterized by exacerbations and remissions. Infrequently, prolonged obstruction can lead to secondary biliary cirrhosis.[100] Hammel and colleagues[101] found regression of liver fibrosis in patients with CP-related CBD strictures after biliary drainage.

Before any treatment, determination of the nature of the stricture is essential, particularly in patients with longstanding CP, because of the possibility of underlying pancreatic cancer, which is increased in such patients. Usually patients with CBD strictures related to CP have simultaneous obstruction of the main pancreatic duct. In these patients, concomitant placement of a plastic pancreatic stent or drainage of a pseudocyst is also performed.[88]

CP-related CBD strictures are much more resistant to endoscopic treatment compared with CBD strictures related to other benign causes.[102,103] Despite the finding that some CP-related CBD strictures may resolve with time, the vast majority should be considered as permanent. Eventually all plastic stents occlude, leading to recurrent signs of biliary obstruction and cholangitis. Consequently, the goal of endoscopic therapy of plastic stent placement in these patients should be carefully evaluated. Definitive therapy of CP-related CBD strictures, especially in younger patients, is surgical drainage by Roux-en-Y hepaticojejunostomy.[88,104]

Endoscopic stent placement of CBD strictures due to CP is indicated in patients who are unfit for surgery because of severe comorbidities or in those who absolutely refuse surgery. Endoscopic plastic stent placement can also be performed as a bridge to surgery in those patients who initially refuse operation, or in cases of severe jaundice when surgery is delayed.

Despite the peribiliary fibrosis, these strictures can be easily traversed with a guidewire and guiding catheter. Placement of 10 or 11.5 French stents is not technically difficult. Balloon dilation before a single stent placement is seldom necessary.

Unfortunately, endoscopic treatment of these strictures with a single plastic stent is effective only in the short-term. Long-term results have been disappointing with recurrence of strictures in 62% to 88% after stent removal (**Table 1**). The presence of calcifications in the pancreatic head parenchyma is associated with a worse response.[105,106] Single plastic stent placement is associated with occlusion (8%–36%), migration (1%–23%), and poor long-term efficacy.[107–112]

A new approach to endoscopic treatment of biliary strictures in the setting of CP is balloon dilation combined with insertion of multiple plastic stents (**Fig. 3**). Draganov and colleagues[113] reported the results of sequential insertion of multiple plastic stents for benign biliary strictures. In this study, 9 patients with CP-related CBD strictures were retrospectively analyzed, and a 44% long-term success rate was achieved (**Table 2**).

In a prospective, nonrandomized trial, Catalano and colleagues[106] compared the use of single and multiple plastic biliary stents in the treatment of patients with CP-related CBD strictures. Long-term results were significantly better in patients treated with multiple stents compared with those treated with single stents (4-year success, 92% vs 24%, respectively; $P<.01$) (see **Table 2**).

Pozsar and colleagues[114] performed a retrospective study of 29 patients with CBD strictures related to CP that underwent biliary stent placement with increasing number of plastic stents. The investigators reported successful long-term outcomes in 60% of patients (see **Table 2**).

Table 1
Summary of series of treatment of common bile duct strictures related to chronic pancreatitis with endoscopic biliary plastic single and multiple stents

Author and Reference	Year	N	Single/Multiple Stents	Long-Term Success (%)	Mean Stenting Duration (Months)	Stent Dysfunction of Any Cause (%)	Follow-up After Stent Removal
Deviere et al[112]	1990	25	Single	12	n/a	72	14
Barthet et al[111]	1994	19	Single	10	10	n/a	18
Smits et al[150]	1996	58	Single	28	10	64	49
Farnbacher et al[110]	2000	31	Single	32	10	52	28
Vitale et al[109]	2000	25	Single	80	13	20	32
Eickoff et al[108]	2001	39	Single	31	9	43	58
Draganov et al[113]	2002	9	Multiple	44	14	n/a	48
Kahl et al[105]	2003	61	Single	26	12	34	40
Catalano et al[106]	2004	34	Single	24	21	41	50
Catalano et al[106]	2004	12	Multiple	92	14	8	47
Pozsar et al[114]	2004	29	Multiple	60	21	n/a	12
Bartoli et al[151]	2005	9	Single	44	9	22	16

Abbreviation: n/a, not available.

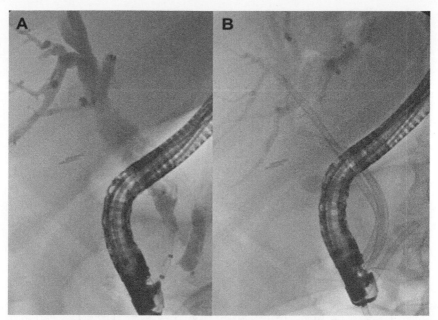

Fig. 3. Endoscopic management of a distal common bile duct stricture caused by chronic pancreatitis. (*A*) ERCP showing a common bile-duct stricture secondary to chronic pancreatitis. (*B*) Three 10-French biliary stents and 1 pancreatic stent were inserted.

Endoscopic treatment of biliary strictures in CP with multiple plastic stent placement may require 1 to 2 years. Similar to the treatment of POBS, stents are exchanged every 3 months, increasing their number at each stent exchange.[106,113,114] The most frequent procedure-related risks of stent placement in this setting are pancreatitis, failed or inadequate positioning (resulting in early cholangitis), migration, perforation, and post-sphincterotomy bleeding. Fatal biliary sepsis caused by stent malfunction has been reported in up to 7% of patients, even in patients with multiple biliary stents.[114]

Progressive dilatation with multiple plastic stents has the disadvantage of requiring multiple procedures. A high rate of complications has been found in noncompliant patients, especially in alcoholics.[107]

Despite some encouraging outcomes, endoscopic biliary plastic stent placement, including multiple stent placement, remains a marginally beneficial therapy for selected patients with chronic pancreatitis who might derive better benefit from permanent surgical biliary bypass. Nevertheless, surgery remains a viable treatment when placement of multiple plastic stents fails.

Recently, self-expandable metal stents have been used to treat CP-related CBD strictures with good outcomes at midterm follow-up, and might be proposed for patients unfit for surgery as a more effective alternative to plastic stent placement.[115–117]

DOMINANT STRICTURES IN PRIMARY SCLEROSING CHOLANGITIS

Plastic stents have been used for the management of dominant biliary strictures in patients with primary sclerosing cholangitis (PSC) with variable results.

PSC is a chronic cholestatic hepatic disease characterized by progressive fibrosing inflammatory involvement of the intrahepatic and extrahepatic bile ducts, leading to

Table 2
Endoscopic treatment of anastomotic biliary strictures in deceased-donor liver transplantation

Study	Number of Patients	Technique	ERCPs/ Patient	Stricture Dilation (%)	Recurrence n (%)	Long-Term Clinical Success (%)	Complications n/ERCPs (%)	Follow-up (Months)
Tabibian et al,[69] 2010	69	Multiple stents (maximum number)	4.1	65/69 (94)	2/65 (3.0)	65/65 (100.0)	4/286 (4)	11
Gomez et al,[41] 2009	27	BD only (9) or single stent (18)	2.0	27/27 (100)	6/27 (22.0)	22/27 (81.5)	9	36
Kulaksiz et al,[68] 2008	19	BD only (10) or 3 stents (9)	5.7	19/19 (100)	3/19 (16.0)	19/19 (100.0)	n/a	18
Elmi and Silverman,[40] 2007	15	Single stent	3.5	13/15 (87)	0	13/13 (100.0)	5/53 (9)	18
Polese et al,[73] 2007	17	BD only (5) or stents (7)	1.7	12/17 (71)	1/12 (8.0)	11/12 (92.0)	1/32 (3)	17
Akay et al,[71] 2006	20	BD only (4) or single stent (11)	0.6	15/20 (75)	7/15 (47.0)	14/15 (93.0)	4/33 (12)	11
Alazmi et al,[77] 2006	148[a]	Multiple stents (maximum number)	3.1	143/148[a] (97)	24/131 (18.0)	131/131[a] (100.0)	n/a	28
Zoepf et al,[67] 2006	25	BD only (9) or multiple stents (16)	4.4	22/25 (88)	9/22 (40.9)	22/22 (100.0)	13/109 (12)	6
Morelli et al,[72] 2003	25	1–3 stents	3.2	22/25 (88)	1/22 (4.5)	20/22 (91.0)	3/79 (4)	54
Rerknimitr et al,[76] 2002	43	Multiple stents (maximum number)	3.6	43/43 (100)	0	43/43 (100.0)	n/a	40
Schwartz et al,[65] 2000	15	BD	1.3	11/15 (73)	3/11 (28.0)	7/11 (64.0)	4/23 (17)	25
Rossi et al,[74] 1998	15	Single stent	n/a	15/15 (100)	2/12 (16.7)	10/12 (83.3)	n/a	12

Abbreviations: BD, balloon dilation; n/a, not assessable.

[a] A total of 148 patients included in the study, 143 underwent successful ERCP, 12 still under treatment, 131 completed dilation treatment.

cholestasis and cirrhosis. The majority of patients with PSC are also affected by inflammatory bowel disease, especially ulcerative colitis. No effective medical therapy has been found for PSC, which may lead to end stage liver disease and need for transplantation. Despite the variability in clinical presentation, endoscopy plays a role in the management of patients with PSC when they present with clinical and biochemical deterioration and severe cholestasis caused by a dominant biliary stricture involving either the CBD or the right or left main intrahepatic ducts.[118] Underlying cholangiocarcinoma needs to be considered in patients with dominant strictures and tissue sampling obtained at the time of endoscopic therapy.

Current knowledge on the role of endoscopic therapy of PSC is based on retrospective studies, small sample sizes, and insufficient documentation of sustained response after treatment. In these patients, the choice of treatment is generally based more on local preference and expertise than on available evidence.

Dominant strictures in symptomatic patients may be treated by balloon dilation or stent placement. The true impact of endoscopic stent placement is uncertain because there are no prospective, randomized controlled trial (RCT) comparing balloon dilation with endoscopic stent placement. The effects of stent placement on survival are also uncertain (**Fig. 4**).

Based upon review of the literature, none of the treatments currently available is definitively effective in the long term. The variability of clinical presentation and natural course of the disease requires treatment to be individualized. Furthermore, the lack of a uniform definition of endoscopic success of PSC-related dominant biliary strictures makes comparison of studies difficult. Finally, the gastroenterological community is divided into stent supporters and stent detractors.[119–123]

In 1996, a European group[120] reported favorable outcomes in 25 patients treated with temporary stent placement. Endoscopic stent placement was technically successful in 21 of 25 patients (84%); patients underwent a median of 3 procedures and were followed for a median of 29 months. Despite the need for retreatment in the majority of patients, the presence of jaundice decreased from 62% to 14%, right upper-quadrant abdominal pain decreased from 52% to 14%, pruritus decreased from 52% to 5%, and fever decreased from 38% to 10%. Complications of ERCP occurred in 14% of procedures and emergency ERCP for stent occlusion was required 32 times.

Because of the high risk of stent occlusion and complication rates, the same group examined a different stent protocol. Dominant strictures were treated with short-term stent placement (mean 11 days). Thirty-two patients were included in a prospective study, and underwent a total of 45 procedures. Two months after short-term stent therapy, cholestatic complaints improved in 83% of patients. Median follow-up was 35 months, and at 1 and 3 years 80% and 60% of patients, respectively, did not require endoscopic reintervention. Mild complications occurred in 15% of patients.[124]

More recently, Gluck and colleagues[119] reported their experience with endoscopic therapy of symptomatic PSC strictures over a 20-year period. Eighty-four patients with dominant strictures underwent 291 ERCPs for acute cholangitis unresponsive to antibiotic treatment, worsening jaundice, pruritus, or pain. Of the 84 patients, 70% had balloon dilations on 1 or more occasions; temporary stents were placed in 51% of patients on 1 or more occasions, usually to facilitate the drainage of infected bile ducts and increase duct patency. ERCP-related complications occurred in 7.2% of procedures and included pancreatitis (3.4%); worsening cholangitis (1%); sepsis (1%); and ductal perforation, bleeding, and liver abscess occurred in a minor percentage. The investigators also evaluated the effects of endoscopic therapy on patient survival, compared with survival predicted by the Mayo Clinic natural-history model. Observed and predicted survival rates were not significantly different for the first 2 years after

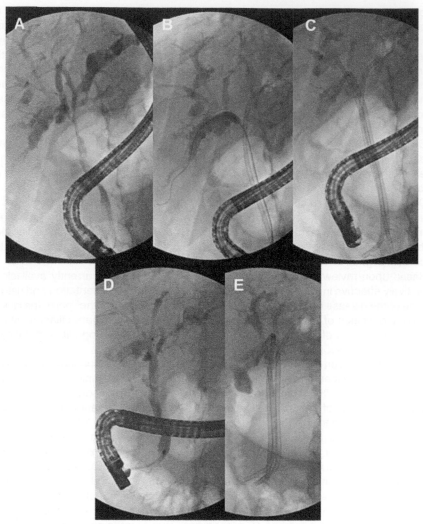

Fig. 4. Endoscopic plastic stent placement in primary sclerosing cholangitis (*A*) ERCP showing diffuse intrahepatic biliary strictures, a dominant stricture at the hilum and another dominant stricture in the CBD (immediately behind the duodenoscope) are present. (*B*) Balloon dilation of the stricture on the right hepatic duct. (*C*) Placement of 3 plastic stents (10 French). (*D*) Four months after stent placement, stricture persists; diffuse irregularity of intrahepatic bile ducts, with sludge and debris. (*E*) After stricture balloon dilation, placement of 4 plastic stents.

treatment, but by year 3 observed survival was statistically higher than predicted survival after stent placement (87% vs 76%).[119]

To the authors' knowledge only 1 study retrospectively compared the outcome of stent placement and balloon dilation in patients with PSC.[121] In this study, 34 patients underwent endoscopic balloon dilation of a dominant stricture (4–8-mm balloons); 19 underwent percutaneous transhepatic stent placement; 14 underwent endoscopic plastic stent placement (7–10 French); and 4 underwent stent placement during PTC and ERCP. Endoscopically placed stents were exchanged every 3 to 4 months.

Complications and cholangitis were significantly more common in the stent group compared with the balloon-dilation group. There were more complications related to percutaneous than endoscopic stent placement (23% vs 7%). However, there was no significant difference between the two groups regarding improving cholestasis and symptom resolution. Despite the relative improvement in jaundice, there was no significant long-term benefit of biliary drainage (either with balloon dilation or stenting) on pruritus or abdominal pain in long-term follow-up.[121] The investigators eventually supported balloon dilation for the management of PSC-associated dominant strictures despite the lack of significant clinical benefits because it was associated with lower complication rates compared with endoscopic stent placement.

Other investigators reported on 500 balloon dilations and 5 stent placements in 96 patients with dominant strictures who were followed for a median period of 7.1 years. Complications rarely occurred and included pancreatitis (2.2%), acute cholangitis (1.4%), and bile duct perforation (0.2%). Endoscopic interventions were repeated over time. However, none of the patients had complete and sustained symptomatic relief or resolution in cholestasis during long-term follow-up. Liver disease eventually led to the need for transplantation in 22.9% of patients. Survival free liver transplantation occurred in 81% after 5 years and 51% after 10 years.[122]

ERCP should be performed carefully and only when strictly indicated in patients with PSC.[123] Severe deterioration of health status has been observed after ERCP, balloon dilation, or stent placement, more likely because of introduction of contamination above strictures in patients with end-stage liver disease.[121]

ACUTE CHOLECYSTITIS AND GALLBLADDER DRAINAGE

The standard of care in operative candidates with acute cholecystitis is urgent laparoscopic cholecystectomy. Laparoscopic cholecystectomy performed within 24 to 72 hours from onset of symptoms is associated with a significantly shortened length of hospital stay than delayed cholecystectomy, whereas operation time, conversion rate, and overall complication rates are not significantly different with the two approaches.[125] However, in a variety of clinical situations (patients with severe cardiopulmonary complications, advanced neoplasms, end-stage liver disease), urgent cholecystectomy may not be advisable because of the high risk, so alternative treatments have been proposed for these patients. Nonoperative gallbladder-drainage techniques include percutaneous gallbladder aspiration, percutaneous cholecystostomy tube placement, and endoscopic transpapillary drainage via nasocystic gallbladder drainage tube or transpapillary stent placement. Recently endoscopic ultrasound–guided transmural gallbladder drainage has been also performed in a small number of patients.[126,127]

Percutaneous gallbladder-drainage techniques have good technical and clinical success rates in patients with acute cholecystitis. However, endoscopic drainage may be preferable to the percutaneous route for a variety of reasons: the external percutaneous tube may be painful and limit daily activities; may prolong hospitalization; and may be associated with a variety of local or general complications, such as cutaneous infections or sepsis.[126]

Endoscopic gallbladder drainage is technically difficult, especially for passage of a guidewire and catheter across the cystic duct. The technical difficulties and the risk of ERCP-related complications have limited the wide use of this method of drainage as first-line nonoperative therapy for acute cholecystitis.

The technique of gallbladder drainage is now standardized.[126,128–140] Most investigators do not recommend routinely performing biliary sphincterotomy.[128,131,134,135,137,139]

However, endoscopic sphincterotomy may be necessary when simultaneous treatment of bile duct stones or biliary strictures is performed. The authors usually perform a biliary sphincterotomy at the time of endoscopic transpapillary gallbladder drainage (**Fig. 5**).[132]

The most challenging part of transpapillary gallbladder drainage is negotiation of the cystic duct with a guidewire. Angled-tip guidewires are preferable to enter into the cystic duct orifice and pass through the spiral valves of the cystic duct while minimizing the risk of perforation. A variety of guidewires have been used. Guidewires can be passed using standard catheters. Sometimes the use of a bendable cannula or a sphincterotome may be of help to enter the cystic duct orifice; the sphincterotome is bowed above the cystic duct insertion and then gently withdrawn until its tip falls into the cystic duct opening. The underlying etiology of acute cholecystitis is often obstruction of the cystic duct by a stone. However, adequate maneuvers with the use of a guidewire and catheter may be effective in disimpaction of the stone into the gallbladder lumen. When the cystic duct has been cannulated, the guidewire has to be passed into the gallbladder lumen. Subsequent placement of a nasocystic gallbladder drain or plastic biliary stent is straightforward, although on occasion the cystic duct needs to be balloon dilated using a 4-mm balloon. Double-pigtail 6 to 10 French-diameter stents are preferable for this clinical application because of their superior anchorage into the gallbladder lumen compared with straight stents. The stent length is chosen based upon the distance between the papilla of Vater and the gallbladder (usually 12–15-cm-long stents are necessary) and the stent size according to the diameter of the cystic duct and CBD (the larger the stent, the longer the patency).

Only retrospective data from referral centers that include small numbers of patients are available on endoscopic gallbladder stent placement (**Table 3**).[128,131–133,135,137–140]

Endoscopic stent placement has been technically successful in the majority of patients in whom it was attempted. A positive clinical response was reported in almost 90% of cases, with few adverse events. When endoscopic gallbladder stent placement was intended as a bridge to surgery, cholecystectomy or liver transplantation were feasible in all cases.[128,131–133,135,137–140]

One of the main concerns with gallbladder stent placement is that acute cholecystitis or sepsis may occur because of stent occlusion.[128,131–133,139] In one study, 8% of patients died of septic shock as a consequence of stent placement.[133]

Indications for endoscopic gallbladder stent placement have not been defined. Endoscopic gallbladder drainage could be attempted in all patients with acute cholecystitis and simultaneous CBD obstruction. Gallbladder stent placement might be also justified in symptomatic patients with end-stage liver disease because percutaneous drainage may be impossible or a high risk in these patients.[131,135,139] Patients awaiting liver transplantation might also benefit from endoscopic stent placement.[135] Finally, the transoral approach might be preferred in patients with severe burns or in those with acalculous cholecystitis in an intensive care unit.

IRRETRIEVABLE BILIARY STONES

Endoscopic removal of common bile duct stones by standard techniques fails in 10% to 20% of cases.[141] These cases are usually treated by large-balloon biliary dilation, mechanical lithotripsy, intraductal shock wave lithotripsy, or extracorporeal shock wave lithotripsy. When these techniques fail, are not available, or cannot be used (ie, patient age, comorbidities, anticoagulation), insertion of a biliary stent to bypass the stone is an effective option (**Fig. 6**). Stone dissolution occurs in more than half of cases within 3 to 6 months and stent placement facilitates removal at subsequent ERCP, making extraction feasible by standard methods.[142–144]

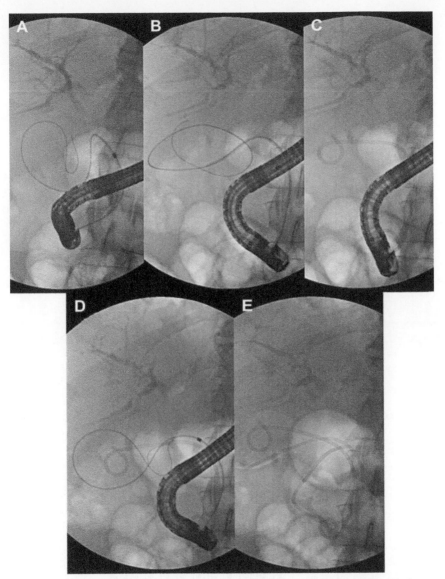

Fig. 5. Endoscopic gallbladder stenting in a patient with acute cholecystitis. (*A*) The cystic duct has been negotiated using a guiding catheter and a hydrophilic guidewire. (*B, C*) A 7-French, double-pigtail plastic stent has been pushed and released between the gall-bladder and the duodenal lumen. (*D*) The cystic duct has been negotiated again with a guidewire. (*E*) Placement of a 6-French naso-gallbladder drainage for flushing the gall-bladder, reducing the risk of stent occlusion and cholecystitis relapse.

Seven- or 10-French straight stents have been used to drain the bile ducts in patients with irretrievable stones. Stents may allow continuous friction on the stone, enhanced by body and intestinal movements.[145] Double-pigtail stents with the prox-imal pigtail wrapped around the stone led to stone dissolution in 70% of cases after 6 months.[145,146] Although addition of oral ursodeoxycholic acid to biliary stenting was not effective in improving stone dissolution in a RCT,[147] the combination

Table 3
Endoscopic transpapillary gallbladder drainage: outcomes of published series

Author	Study Design	Number of Patients	Acute Cholecystitis (%)	Technical Success (%)	Clinical Response (Stent Successfully Placed) (%)	Follow-up (Months)	Recurrences
Tamada et al,[140] 1991	Retrospective	14	100	n/a	64	2	0/14
Kalloo et al,[137] 1994	Retrospective	4	25	100	100	11–17	0/4
Gaglio et al,[138] 1996	Retrospective	3	100	n/a	100	4–6	2/3
Shrestha et al,[135] 1999	Prospective	13	54	100	100	1–36	1/12
Conway et al,[139] 2005	Retrospective	29	23	90	96	9	2/26
Schlenker et al,[131] 2006	Retrospective	23	48	100	78	2–54	3/18
Pannala et al,[133] 2008	Retrospective	51[a]	78	100	98	n/a	n/a
Mutignani et al,[132] 2009	Retrospective	35[a]	100	83	83	17	4/17
Lee et al,[128] 2011	Prospective	23	91	79	100	20	2/20

[a] Including cases of naso-gallbladder drainage.

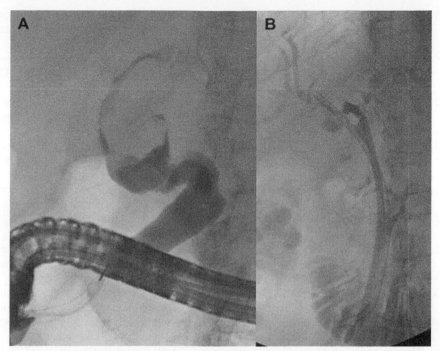

Fig. 6. Plastic stent placement for the management of irretrievable biliary stone. (*A*) A huge common bile duct stone in an 82-year-old woman with several comorbidities. (*B*) Two 10-French stents were inserted to bypass the stone with good contrast drainage.

of ursodeoxycholic acid, terpene preparation, and biliary stent placement might increase the stone dissolution rate.[144,148]

An attempt at stone extraction is suggested within 3 to 6 months of stent insertion because death caused by stent-related cholangitis has been reported in up to 6.7% to 16.0% after a stent has been left in place long-term.[149]

REFERENCES

1. Soehendra N, Reynders-Frederix V. [Palliative biliary duct drainage. A new method for endoscopic introduction of a new drain]. Dtsch Med Wochenschr 1979;104:206–7 [in German].
2. Bjorkman DJ, Carr-Locke DL, Lichtenstein DR, et al. Postsurgical bile leaks: endoscopic obliteration of the transpapillary pressure gradient is enough. Am J Gastroenterol 1995;90:2128–33.
3. Chow S, Bosco JJ, Heiss FW, et al. Successful treatment of post-cholecystectomy bile leaks using nasobiliary tube drainage and sphincterotomy. Am J Gastroenterol 1997;92:1839–43.
4. Sugiyama M, Mori T, Atomi Y. Endoscopic nasobiliary drainage for treating bile leak after laparoscopic cholecystectomy. Hepatogastroenterology 1999;46:762–5.
5. Saab S, Martin P, Soliman GY, et al. Endoscopic management of biliary leaks after T-tube removal in liver transplant recipients: nasobiliary drainage versus biliary stenting. Liver Transpl 2000;6:627–32.

6. Binmoeller KF, Katon RM, Shneidman R. Endoscopic management of postoperative biliary leaks: review of 77 cases and report of two cases with biloma formation. Am J Gastroenterol 1991;86:227–31.

7. Marks JM, Ponsky JL, Shillingstad RB, et al. Biliary stenting is more effective than sphincterotomy in the resolution of biliary leaks. Surg Endosc 1998;12: 327–30.

8. Pfau PR, Kochman ML, Lewis JD, et al. Endoscopic management of postoperative biliary complications in orthotopic liver transplantation. Gastrointest Endosc 2000;52:55–63.

9. Morelli J, Mulcahy HE, Willner IR, et al. Endoscopic treatment of post-liver transplantation biliary leaks with stent placement across the leak site. Gastrointest Endosc 2001;54:471–5.

10. Shah JN. Endoscopic treatment of bile leaks: current standards and recent innovations. Gastrointest Endosc 2007;65:1069–72.

11. Llach J, Bordas JM, Elizalde JI, et al. Sphincterotomy in the treatment of biliary leakage. Hepatogastroenterology 2002;49:1496–8.

12. Sandha GS, Bourke MJ, Haber GB, et al. Endoscopic therapy for bile leak based on a new classification: results in 207 patients. Gastrointest Endosc 2004;60:567–74.

13. Mavrogiannis C, Liatsos C, Papanikolaou IS, et al. Biliary stenting alone versus biliary stenting plus sphincterotomy for the treatment of post-laparoscopic cholecystectomy biliary leaks: a prospective randomized study. Eur J Gastroenterol Hepatol 2006;18:405–9.

14. Katsinelos P, Kountouras J, Paroutoglou G, et al. A comparative study of 10-Fr vs. 7-Fr straight plastic stents in the treatment of postcholecystectomy bile leak. Surg Endosc 2008;22:101–6.

15. Aksoz K, Unsal B, Yoruk G, et al. Endoscopic sphincterotomy alone in the management of low-grade biliary leaks due to cholecystectomy. Dig Endosc 2009;21:158–61.

16. Mergener K, Strobel JC, Suhocki P, et al. The role of ERCP in diagnosis and management of accessory bile duct leaks after cholecystectomy. Gastrointest Endosc 1999;50:527–31.

17. Mutignani M, Shah SK, Tringali A, et al. Endoscopic therapy for biliary leaks from aberrant right hepatic ducts severed during cholecystectomy. Gastrointest Endosc 2002;55:932–6.

18. Bismuth H, Majno PE. Biliary strictures: classification based on the principles of surgical treatment. World J Surg 2001;25:1241–4.

19. Sicklick JK, Camp MS, Lillemoe KD, et al. Surgical management of bile duct injuries sustained during laparoscopic cholecystectomy: perioperative results in 200 patients. Ann Surg 2005;241:786–92.

20. Sikora SS, Pottakkat B, Srikanth G, et al. Postcholecystectomy benign biliary strictures - long-term results. Dig Surg 2006;23:304–12.

21. Walsh RM, Henderson JM, Vogt DP, et al. Long-term outcome of biliary reconstruction for bile duct injuries from laparoscopic cholecystectomies. Surgery 2007;142:450–6.

22. Nuzzo G, Giuliante F, Giovannini I, et al. Advantages of multidisciplinary management of bile duct injuries occurring during cholecystectomy. Am J Surg 2008;195:763–9.

23. Bergman JJ, Burgemeister L, Bruno MJ, et al. Long-term follow-up after biliary stent placement for postoperative bile duct stenosis. Gastrointest Endosc 2001; 54:154–61.

24. Costamagna G, Pandolfi M, Mutignani M, et al. Long-term results of endoscopic management of postoperative bile duct strictures with increasing numbers of stents. Gastrointest Endosc 2001;54:162–8.
25. Costamagna G, Tringali A, Mutignani M, et al. Endotherapy of postoperative biliary strictures with multiple stents: results after more than 10 years of follow-up. Gastrointest Endosc 2010;72:551–7.
26. Kuzela L, Oltman M, Sutka J, et al. Prospective follow-up of patients with bile duct strictures secondary to laparoscopic cholecystectomy, treated endoscopically with multiple stents. Hepatogastroenterology 2005;52:1357–61.
27. Zajko AB, Campbell WL, Bron KM, et al. Diagnostic and interventional radiology in liver transplantation. Gastroenterol Clin North Am 1988;17:105–43.
28. Weber A, Prinz C, Gerngross C, et al. Long-term outcome of endoscopic and/or percutaneous transhepatic therapy in patients with biliary stricture after orthotopic liver transplantation. J Gastroenterol 2009;44:1195–202.
29. Colonna JO, Shaked A, Gomes AS, et al. Biliary strictures complicating liver transplantation. Incidence, pathogenesis, management, and outcome. Ann Surg 1992;216:344–50.
30. Balderramo D, Navasa M, Cardenas A. Current management of biliary complications after liver transplantation: emphasis on endoscopic therapy. Gastroenterol Hepatol 2011;34:107–15.
31. Williams ED, Draganov PV. Endoscopic management of biliary strictures after liver transplantation. World J Gastroenterol 2009;15:3725–33.
32. Londono MC, Balderramo D, Cardenas A. Management of biliary complications after orthotopic liver transplantation: the role of endoscopy. World J Gastroenterol 2008;14:493–7.
33. Graziadei IW, Schwaighofer H, Koch R, et al. Long-term outcome of endoscopic treatment of biliary strictures after liver transplantation. Liver Transpl 2006;12: 718–25.
34. Verdonk RC, Buis CI, Porte RJ, et al. Biliary complications after liver transplantation: a review. Scand J Gastroenterol Suppl 2006;(243):89–101.
35. Thuluvath PJ, Pfau PR, Kimmey MB, et al. Biliary complications after liver transplantation: the role of endoscopy. Endoscopy 2005;37:857–63.
36. Pascher A, Neuhaus P. Bile duct complications after liver transplantation. Transpl Int 2005;18:627–42.
37. Alawi K, Khalaf H, Medhat Y, et al. Risk factors for biliary complications after living-donor liver transplant: a single-center experience. Exp Clin Transplant 2008;6:101–4.
38. Chang JH, Lee IS, Choi JY, et al. Biliary stricture after adult right-lobe living-donor liver transplantation with duct-to-duct anastomosis: long-term outcome and its related factors after endoscopic treatment. Gut Liver 2010;4:226–33.
39. Dorobantu B, Brasoveanu V, Matei E, et al. Biliary complications after liver transplantation–523 consecutive cases in two centers. Hepatogastroenterology 2010;57:932–8.
40. Elmi F, Silverman WB. Outcome of ERCP in the management of duct-to-duct anastomotic strictures in orthotopic liver transplant. Dig Dis Sci 2007;52:2346–50.
41. Gomez CM, Dumonceau JM, Marcolongo M, et al. Endoscopic management of biliary complications after adult living-donor versus deceased-donor liver transplantation. Transplantation 2009;88:1280–5.
42. Hintze RE, Adler A, Veltzke W, et al. Endoscopic management of biliary complications after orthotopic liver transplantation. Hepatogastroenterology 1997;44: 258–62.

43. Kato H, Kawamoto H, Tsutsumi K, et al. Long-term outcomes of endoscopic management for biliary strictures after living donor liver transplantation with duct-to-duct reconstruction. Transpl Int 2009;22:914–21.

44. Kohler S, Pascher A, Mittler J, et al. Management of biliary complications following living donor liver transplantation–a single center experience. Langenbecks Arch Surg 2009;394:1025–31.

45. Macfarlane B, Davidson B, Dooley JS, et al. Endoscopic retrograde cholangiography in the diagnosis and endoscopic management of biliary complications after liver transplantation. Eur J Gastroenterol Hepatol 1996;8:1003–6.

46. Mosca S, Militerno G, Guardascione MA, et al. Late biliary tract complications after orthotopic liver transplantation: diagnostic and therapeutic role of endoscopic retrograde cholangiopancreatography. J Gastroenterol Hepatol 2000; 15:654–60.

47. Saidi RF, Elias N, Ko DS, et al. Biliary reconstruction and complications after living-donor liver transplantation. HPB (Oxford) 2009;11:505–9.

48. Sanna C, Saracco GM, Reggio D, et al. Endoscopic retrograde cholangiopancreatography in patients with biliary complications after orthotopic liver transplantation: outcomes and complications. Transplant Proc 2009;41:1319–21.

49. Seo JK, Ryu JK, Lee SH, et al. Endoscopic treatment for biliary stricture after adult living donor liver transplantation. Liver Transpl 2009;15:369–80.

50. Shah SA, Grant DR, McGilvray ID, et al. Biliary strictures in 130 consecutive right lobe living donor liver transplant recipients: results of a Western center. Am J Transplant 2007;7:161–7.

51. Tashiro H, Itamoto T, Sasaki T, et al. Biliary complications after duct-to-duct biliary reconstruction in living-donor liver transplantation: causes and treatment. World J Surg 2007;31:2222–9.

52. Tsujino T, Isayama H, Sugawara Y, et al. Endoscopic management of biliary complications after adult living donor liver transplantation. Am J Gastroenterol 2006;101:2230–6.

53. Yazumi S, Yoshimoto T, Hisatsune H, et al. Endoscopic treatment of biliary complications after right-lobe living-donor liver transplantation with duct-to-duct biliary anastomosis. J Hepatobiliary Pancreat Surg 2006;13:502–10.

54. Zoepf T, Maldonado-Lopez EJ, Hilgard P, et al. Endoscopic therapy of post-transplant biliary stenoses after right-sided adult living donor liver transplantation. Clin Gastroenterol Hepatol 2005;3:1144–9.

55. Buis CI, Geuken E, Visser DS, et al. Altered bile composition after liver transplantation is associated with the development of nonanastomotic biliary strictures. J Hepatol 2009;50:69–79.

56. Lee HW, Suh KS, Shin WY, et al. Classification and prognosis of intrahepatic biliary stricture after liver transplantation. Liver Transpl 2007;13:1736–42.

57. Buis CI, Verdonk RC, van der Jagt EJ, et al. Nonanastomotic biliary strictures after liver transplantation, part 1: radiological features and risk factors for early vs. late presentation. Liver Transpl 2007;13:708–18.

58. Verdonk RC, Buis CI, van der Jagt EJ, et al. Nonanastomotic biliary strictures after liver transplantation, part 2: management, outcome, and risk factors for disease progression. Liver Transpl 2007;13:725–32.

59. Farid WR, de JJ, Slieker JC, et al. The importance of portal venous blood flow in ischemic-type biliary lesions after liver transplantation. Am J Transplant 2011;11:857–62.

60. Foley DP, Fernandez LA, Leverson G, et al. Donation after cardiac death: the University of Wisconsin experience with liver transplantation. Ann Surg 2005; 242:724–31.

61. Sanchez-Urdazpal L, Gores GJ, Ward EM, et al. Ischemic-type biliary complications after orthotopic liver transplantation. Hepatology 1992;16:49–53.
62. Chahal P, Baron TH, Poterucha JJ, et al. Endoscopic retrograde cholangiography in post-orthotopic liver transplant population with Roux-en-Y biliary reconstruction. Liver Transpl 2007;13:1168–73.
63. Haruta H, Yamamoto H, Mizuta K, et al. A case of successful enteroscopic balloon dilation for late anastomotic stricture of choledochojejunostomy after living donor liver transplantation. Liver Transpl 2005;11:1608–10.
64. Baron TH. Establishing a systematic endoscopic approach to the management of anastomotic biliary strictures is needed. Liver Transpl 2001;7:378–9.
65. Schwartz DA, Petersen BT, Poterucha JJ, et al. Endoscopic therapy of anastomotic bile duct strictures occurring after liver transplantation. Gastrointest Endosc 2000;51:169–74.
66. Mahajani RV, Cotler SJ, Uzer MF. Efficacy of endoscopic management of anastomotic biliary strictures after hepatic transplantation. Endoscopy 2000;32:943–9.
67. Zoepf T, Maldonado-Lopez EJ, Hilgard P, et al. Balloon dilatation vs. balloon dilatation plus bile duct endoprostheses for treatment of anastomotic biliary strictures after liver transplantation. Liver Transpl 2006;12:88–94.
68. Kulaksiz H, Weiss KH, Gotthardt D, et al. Is stenting necessary after balloon dilation of post-transplantation biliary strictures? Results of a prospective comparative study. Endoscopy 2008;40:746–51.
69. Tabibian JH, Asham EH, Han S, et al. Endoscopic treatment of postorthotopic liver transplantation anastomotic biliary strictures with maximal stent therapy (with video). Gastrointest Endosc 2010;71:505–12.
70. St Peter S, Rodriquez-Davalos MI, Rodriguez-Luna HM, et al. Significance of proximal biliary dilatation in patients with anastomotic strictures after liver transplantation. Dig Dis Sci 2004;49:1207–11.
71. Akay S, Karasu Z, Ersoz G, et al. Results of endoscopic management of anastomotic biliary strictures after orthotopic liver transplantation. Turk J Gastroenterol 2006;17:159–63.
72. Morelli J, Mulcahy HE, Willner IR, et al. Long-term outcomes for patients with post-liver transplant anastomotic biliary strictures treated by endoscopic stent placement. Gastrointest Endosc 2003;58:374–9.
73. Polese L, Cillo U, Brolese A, et al. Endoscopic treatment of bile duct complications after orthotopic liver transplantation. Transplant Proc 2007;39:1942–4.
74. Rossi AF, Grosso C, Zanasi G, et al. Long-term efficacy of endoscopic stenting in patients with stricture of the biliary anastomosis after orthotopic liver transplantation. Endoscopy 1998;30:360–6.
75. Solmi L, Cariani G, Leo P, et al. Results of endoscopic retrograde cholangiopancreatography in the treatment of biliary tract complications after orthotopic liver transplantation: our experience. Hepatogastroenterology 2007;54:1004–8.
76. Rerknimitr R, Sherman S, Fogel EL, et al. Biliary tract complications after orthotopic liver transplantation with choledochocholedochostomy anastomosis: endoscopic findings and results of therapy. Gastrointest Endosc 2002;55:224–31.
77. Alazmi WM, Fogel EL, Watkins JL, et al. Recurrence rate of anastomotic biliary strictures in patients who have had previous successful endoscopic therapy for anastomotic narrowing after orthotopic liver transplantation. Endoscopy 2006;38:571–4.
78. Morelli G, Fazel A, Judah J, et al. Rapid-sequence endoscopic management of posttransplant anastomotic biliary strictures. Gastrointest Endosc 2008;67:879–85.

79. Tabibian JH, Asham EH, Goldstein L, et al. Endoscopic treatment with multiple stents for post-liver-transplantation nonanastomotic biliary strictures. Gastrointest Endosc 2009;69:1236–43.

80. Ward EM, Kiely MJ, Maus TP, et al. Hilar biliary strictures after liver transplantation: cholangiography and percutaneous treatment. Radiology 1990;177:259–63.

81. Rizk RS, McVicar JP, Emond MJ, et al. Endoscopic management of biliary strictures in liver transplant recipients: effect on patient and graft survival. Gastrointest Endosc 1998;47:128–35.

82. Duailibi DF, Ribeiro MA Jr. Biliary complications following deceased and living donor liver transplantation: a review. Transplant Proc 2010;42:517–20.

83. Egawa H, Inomata Y, Uemoto S, et al. Biliary anastomotic complications in 400 living related liver transplantations. World J Surg 2001;25:1300–7.

84. Tsujino T, Sugawara Y, Omata M. Management of biliary strictures after living donor liver transplantation. Gastrointest Endosc 2009;70:599–600.

85. Hisatsune H, Yazumi S, Egawa H, et al. Endoscopic management of biliary strictures after duct-to-duct biliary reconstruction in right-lobe living-donor liver transplantation. Transplantation 2003;76:810–5.

86. Kim TH, Lee SK, Han JH, et al. The role of endoscopic retrograde cholangiography for biliary stricture after adult living donor liver transplantation: technical aspect and outcome. Scand J Gastroenterol 2011;46:188–96.

87. Shah JN, Ahmad NA, Shetty K, et al. Endoscopic management of biliary complications after adult living donor liver transplantation. Am J Gastroenterol 2004;99:1291–5.

88. Adler DG, Lichtenstein D, Baron TH, et al. The role of endoscopy in patients with chronic pancreatitis. Gastrointest Endosc 2006;63:933–7.

89. Petrozza JA, Dutta SK. The variable appearance of distal common bile duct stenosis in chronic pancreatitis. J Clin Gastroenterol 1985;7:447–50.

90. Sand JA, Nordback IH. Management of cholestasis in patients with chronic pancreatitis: evaluation of a treatment protocol. Eur J Surg 1995;161:587–92.

91. Wislooff F, Jakobsen J, Osnes M. Stenosis of the common bile duct in chronic pancreatitis. Br J Surg 1982;69:52–4.

92. Afroudakis A, Kaplowitz N. Liver histopathology in chronic common bile duct stenosis due to chronic alcoholic pancreatitis. Hepatology 1981;1:65–72.

93. Aranha GV, Prinz RA, Freeark RJ, et al. The spectrum of biliary tract obstruction from chronic pancreatitis. Arch Surg 1984;119:595–600.

94. Huizinga WK, Thomson SR, Spitaels JM, et al. Chronic pancreatitis with biliary obstruction. Ann R Coll Surg Engl 1992;74:119–23.

95. Stabile BE, Calabria R, Wilson SE, et al. Stricture of the common bile duct from chronic pancreatitis. Surg Gynecol Obstet 1987;165:121–6.

96. Yadegar J, Williams RA, Passaro E Jr, et al. Common duct stricture from chronic pancreatitis. Arch Surg 1980;115:582–6.

97. Scott J, Summerfield JA, Elias E, et al. Chronic pancreatitis: a cause of cholestasis. Gut 1977;18:196–201.

98. Sarles H, Sahel J. Cholestasis and lesions of the biliary tract in chronic pancreatitis. Gut 1978;19:851–7.

99. Delhaye M, Arvanitakis M, Bali M, et al. Endoscopic therapy for chronic pancreatitis. Scand J Surg 2005;94:143–53.

100. Abdallah AA, Krige JE, Bornman PC. Biliary tract obstruction in chronic pancreatitis. HPB (Oxford) 2007;9:421–8.

101. Hammel P, Couvelard A, O'Toole D, et al. Regression of liver fibrosis after biliary drainage in patients with chronic pancreatitis and stenosis of the common bile duct. N Engl J Med 2001;344:418–23.

102. Mahajan A, Ho H, Sauer B, et al. Temporary placement of fully covered self-expandable metal stents in benign biliary strictures: midterm evaluation (with video). Gastrointest Endosc 2009;70:303–9.
103. Kahaleh M, Behm B, Clarke BW, et al. Temporary placement of covered self-expandable metal stents in benign biliary strictures: a new paradigm? (with video). Gastrointest Endosc 2008;67:446–54.
104. Nealon WH, Urrutia F. Long-term follow-up after bilioenteric anastomosis for benign bile duct stricture. Ann Surg 1996;223:639–45.
105. Kahl S, Zimmermann S, Genz I, et al. Risk factors for failure of endoscopic stenting of biliary strictures in chronic pancreatitis: a prospective follow-up study. Am J Gastroenterol 2003;98:2448–53.
106. Catalano MF, Linder JD, George S, et al. Treatment of symptomatic distal common bile duct stenosis secondary to chronic pancreatitis: comparison of single vs. multiple simultaneous stents. Gastrointest Endosc 2004;60:945–52.
107. Kiehne K, Folsch UR, Nitsche R. High complication rate of bile duct stents in patients with chronic alcoholic pancreatitis due to noncompliance. Endoscopy 2000;32:377–80.
108. Eickhoff A, Jakobs R, Leonhardt A, et al. Endoscopic stenting for common bile duct stenoses in chronic pancreatitis: results and impact on long-term outcome. Eur J Gastroenterol Hepatol 2001;13:1161–7.
109. Vitale GC, Reed DN Jr, Nguyen CT, et al. Endoscopic treatment of distal bile duct stricture from chronic pancreatitis. Surg Endosc 2000;14:227–31.
110. Farnbacher MJ, Rabenstein T, Ell C, et al. Is endoscopic drainage of common bile duct stenoses in chronic pancreatitis up-to-date? Am J Gastroenterol 2000;95:1466–71.
111. Barthet M, Bernard JP, Duval JL, et al. Biliary stenting in benign biliary stenosis complicating chronic calcifying pancreatitis. Endoscopy 1994;26:569–72.
112. Deviere J, Devaere S, Baize M, et al. Endoscopic biliary drainage in chronic pancreatitis. Gastrointest Endosc 1990;36:96–100.
113. Draganov P, Hoffman B, Marsh W, et al. Long-term outcome in patients with benign biliary strictures treated endoscopically with multiple stents. Gastrointest Endosc 2002;55:680–6.
114. Pozsar J, Sahin P, Laszlo F, et al. Medium-term results of endoscopic treatment of common bile duct strictures in chronic calcifying pancreatitis with increasing numbers of stents. J Clin Gastroenterol 2004;38:118–23.
115. Behm B, Brock A, Clarke BW, et al. Partially covered self-expandable metallic stents for benign biliary strictures due to chronic pancreatitis. Endoscopy 2009;41:547–51.
116. Cahen DL, Rauws EA, Gouma DJ, et al. Removable fully covered self-expandable metal stents in the treatment of common bile duct strictures due to chronic pancreatitis: a case series. Endoscopy 2008;40:697–700.
117. Park do H, Kim MH, Moon SH, et al. Feasibility and safety of placement of a newly designed, fully covered self-expandable metal stent for refractory benign pancreatic ductal strictures: a pilot study (with video). Gastrointest Endosc 2008;68:1182–9.
118. Silveira MG, Lindor KD. Clinical features and management of primary sclerosing cholangitis. World J Gastroenterol 2008;14:3338–49.
119. Gluck M, Cantone NR, Brandabur JJ, et al. A twenty-year experience with endoscopic therapy for symptomatic primary sclerosing cholangitis. J Clin Gastroenterol 2008;42:1032–9.

120. van Milligen de Wit AW, van BJ, Rauws EA, et al. Endoscopic stent therapy for dominant extrahepatic bile duct strictures in primary sclerosing cholangitis. Gastrointest Endosc 1996;44:293–9.
121. Kaya M, Petersen BT, Angulo P, et al. Balloon dilation compared to stenting of dominant strictures in primary sclerosing cholangitis. Am J Gastroenterol 2001;96:1059–66.
122. Gotthardt DN, Rudolph G, Kloters-Plachky P, et al. Endoscopic dilation of dominant stenoses in primary sclerosing cholangitis: outcome after long-term treatment. Gastrointest Endosc 2010;71:527–34.
123. Al-Kawas FH. Endoscopic management of primary sclerosing cholangitis: less is better! Am J Gastroenterol 1999;94:2235–6.
124. Ponsioen CY, Lam K, van Milligen de Wit AW, et al. Four years experience with short term stenting in primary sclerosing cholangitis. Am J Gastroenterol 1999; 94:2403–7.
125. Lau H, Lo CY, Patil NG, et al. Early versus delayed-interval laparoscopic cholecystectomy for acute cholecystitis: a meta-analysis. Surg Endosc 2006;20:82–7.
126. Itoi T, Coelho-Prabhu N, Baron TH. Endoscopic gallbladder drainage for management of acute cholecystitis. Gastrointest Endosc 2010;71:1038–45.
127. Baron TH, Topazian MD. Endoscopic transduodenal drainage of the gallbladder: implications for endoluminal treatment of gallbladder disease. Gastrointest Endosc 2007;65:735–7.
128. Lee TH, Park DH, Lee SS, et al. Outcomes of endoscopic transpapillary gallbladder stenting for symptomatic gallbladder diseases: a multicenter prospective follow-up study*. Endoscopy 2011. [Epub ahead of print].
129. Itoi T, Sofuni A, Itokawa F, et al. Endoscopic transpapillary gallbladder drainage in patients with acute cholecystitis in whom percutaneous transhepatic approach is contraindicated or anatomically impossible (with video). Gastrointest Endosc 2008;68:455–60.
130. Kjaer DW, Kruse A, Funch-Jensen P. Endoscopic gallbladder drainage of patients with acute cholecystitis. Endoscopy 2007;39:304–8.
131. Schlenker C, Trotter JF, Shah RJ, et al. Endoscopic gallbladder stent placement for treatment of symptomatic cholelithiasis in patients with end-stage liver disease. Am J Gastroenterol 2006;101:278–83.
132. Mutignani M, Iacopini F, Perri V, et al. Endoscopic gallbladder drainage for acute cholecystitis: technical and clinical results. Endoscopy 2009;41:539–46.
133. Pannala R, Petersen BT, Gostout CJ, et al. Endoscopic transpapillary gallbladder drainage: 10-year single center experience. Minerva Gastroenterol Dietol 2008;54:107–13.
134. Johlin FC Jr, Neil GA. Drainage of the gallbladder in patients with acute acalculous cholecystitis by transpapillary endoscopic cholecystotomy. Gastrointest Endosc 1993;39:645–51.
135. Shrestha R, Trouillot TE, Everson GT. Endoscopic stenting of the gallbladder for symptomatic gallbladder disease in patients with end-stage liver disease awaiting orthotopic liver transplantation. Liver Transpl Surg 1999;5:275–81.
136. Feretis C, Apostolidis N, Mallas E, et al. Endoscopic drainage of acute obstructive cholecystitis in patients with increased operative risk. Endoscopy 1993;25:392–5.
137. Kalloo AN, Thuluvath PJ, Pasricha PJ. Treatment of high-risk patients with symptomatic cholelithiasis by endoscopic gallbladder stenting. Gastrointest Endosc 1994;40:608–10.

Plastic Biliary Stents for Malignant Biliary Diseases

Inge Huibregtse, MD, PhD, Paul Fockens, MD, PhD*

KEYWORDS

• Malignant • Biliary • Plastic stent • Occlusion

Several malignancies can cause biliary obstruction at different levels with resultant jaundice. These malignancies include carcinoma of the papilla of Vater, pancreatic cancer, gallbladder cancer, distal cholangiocarcinoma, proximal cholangiocarcinoma (also known as Klatskin tumors), and metastatic disease involving pancreatic head and liver hilus. However, obstructive jaundice is often a manifestation of advanced disease, and curative surgery is often not possible. Consequently, palliative relief of common bile duct obstruction is an important part of patient management. Biliary stents can be placed not only to relieve obstructive jaundice for palliative treatment but also for preoperative biliary decompression. Endoscopic biliary stenting is now a well-established palliative treatment modality, and because of its lower risk and cost, this technique has almost completely replaced palliative surgery.[1,2] Plastic endoscopic biliary prostheses were first used to treat malignant obstruction in 1979.[3] Initially, 7F gauge plastic stents were used, but subsequently 10F stents were found to provide longer patency. Over the years, stents of different plastic materials, such as polyethylene, polyurethane, and polytetrafluoroethylene (Teflon), have been used. All plastic biliary stents clog within a few months after insertion (**Fig. 1**). In the late 1980s, uncovered (bare metal) self-expandable metal endoprostheses were introduced. The larger-diameter metal stents still occlude because of tumor ingrowth and/or overgrowth. Furthermore, these uncovered metal stents cannot be removed endoscopically. More recently, fully covered expandable metals stents have become available, which although not designed for removability, can often be endoscopically removed. In this review, the authors discuss the history of plastic biliary stent development and the current use of plastic stents for malignant biliary diseases.

HISTORY

The first endoscopic biliary stent was placed in 1979, an intervention that had been thought to be impossible. In those days, the instrumentation channel of the available

Department of Gastroenterology and Hepatology, Academic Medical Center, University of Amsterdam, PO Box 22700, 1100 DE, Amsterdam, The Netherlands
* Corresponding author.
E-mail address: p.fockens@amc.nl

Gastrointest Endoscopy Clin N Am 21 (2011) 435–445
doi:10.1016/j.giec.2011.04.010
1052-5157/11/$ – see front matter © 2011 Elsevier Inc. All rights reserved.

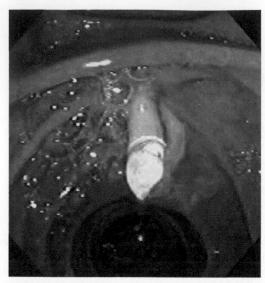

Fig. 1. Occluded 10F stent exiting the bile duct. (*From* Baron TH, Ponsky JL. Plastic pancreatic and biliary stents: concepts and insertion techniques. In: Baron TH, editor. ERCP. Elsevier; 2008. p. 153–63; with permission.)

duodenoscopes only allowed for the insertion of a 7F catheter.[3] The guidewires were at that time rather stiff and had a rough surface, which made stent placement technically difficult. The first endoprosthesis was cut off from an angiographic pigtail catheter. The high incidence of recurrent cholangitis in the first patients treated suggested that hindrance of bile flow in the stent caused occlusion, and the development of larger-diameter stents was deemed necessary. In 1981, Huibregtse and colleagues[4] from the Amsterdam group were the first to describe the insertion of a newly developed straight 10F endoprosthesis with side flaps on both ends, which was passed through a forward-viewing large-channel gastroscope. The significantly prolonged patency and improved outcomes using these larger-diameter stents prompted development of side-viewing endoscopes with a larger-diameter working channel to allow insertion of a 10F endoprosthesis. In April 1981, the first prototype duodenoscope with a 3.7-mm channel was tested. In 1982, the first series of 30 patients with distal malignant biliary obstruction who underwent endoscopic insertion of a 10F stent was published.[5] The technical success rate of endoscopic biliary stenting in distal and mid–common bile duct strictures improved and now exceeds 90% with low insertion-related complication rates. Over time, different stent diameters were tested, ranging from 7F to 12F.[6] Any further increase in stent diameter longer than 10F to 11.5F or even 12F increased the technical difficulty of stent placement without improving stent patency.[7–9] Therefore, a diameter of 10F is thought to be the best combination of patency and technically easy placement.

PLASTIC STENTS

When designing plastic stents, an endoprosthesis should ideally have all of the following characteristics: should be technically easy to insert, should effectively relieve biliary obstruction, should not occlude, and should not cause injury to the bile duct or duodenal wall. Several different materials, sizes, and shapes have been used to try and optimize these aspects. Different materials, such as polyethylene, polyurethane, and polytetrafluoroethylene (Teflon), have been used. In vitro studies showed a direct relation between the coefficient of friction and the amount of encrusted material within the stent lumen. Although Teflon had the lowest friction coefficient and greatest potential for prevention of clogging,[10] it made the endoprostheses stiffer and a higher perforation risk was reported. Polyurethane tubing was also used but became brittle over time. Polyurethane endoprostheses fragmented during attempted retrieval, making removal difficult or even impossible. Polyethylene remains the preferred tubing material because it combines strength with relative softness, making injuries to the bile duct or duodenal wall rare. Although polyethylene has a higher coefficient of friction than Teflon, equal stent patency has been demonstrated.[11] However, results from a meta-analysis showed that polyethylene stents provided superior patency in distal malignant biliary strictures.[1]

Scanning electron microscopy of out-of-package biliary stents has shown that the inner surface smoothness of plastic stents is highly variable, which is probably inherent to the manufacturing process. The smoothness of the stent surface is considered to be an important factor in the occurrence of stent dysfunction.[12] Scanning electron microscopy has shown that polyethylene stents have surface projections, whereas Teflon stents have the most irregular inner surface of all stents with multiple shallow pits and ridges.[13] Only polyurethane stents were found to have a smooth surface.

The first endoprosthesis used for transpapillary endoscopic drainage had multiple side holes and measured 20 cm in length. The excessive length led to premature clogging and damage to the wall of the bile duct or duodenum. Shortening of the endoprosthesis led to a high incidence of proximal stent migration above the stricture. Placement of a second pigtail on the distal end prevented proximal migration, but the incidence of later cholangitis because of stent occlusion remained high. Thus, pigtail stents were replaced by straight endoprostheses with proximal and distal side flaps to prevent migration. These straight endoprosthesis were also easier to introduce. Most plastic stents are slightly curved to contour to the common bile duct (**Fig. 2**). Multiple side holes at both ends of some stents maintain drainage even when the tip of the stent is impacted into the biliary or duodenal wall.

In 1995, a novel straight Teflon stent without side holes called the Tannenbaum prosthesis was introduced. This stent was designed because studies had shown that considerable sludge formation occurred around the side holes of straight stents. Furthermore, at that time, Teflon was thought to have the lowest friction coefficient. Initially, encouraging results were presented in a prospective nonrandomized study, but these results could not be confirmed in subsequent studies comparing the Tannenbaum and polyethylene stents.[14,15] The addition of side holes to Tannenbaum stents, or a stainless steel mesh with polyamide outer layer, did not improve patency compared with standard polyethylene stents.

More recently, 2 stent designs have been used in an attempt to prolong patency of plastic stents. One is the use of a star-shaped stent with a limited central lumen.[16] The other is the addition of an antireflux valve to prevent stent occlusion because of food and vegetable materials.[17] Thus far, these stents have not definitively proven superior patency as compared with traditional plastic stents.[2]

Plastic stents are typically available in lengths ranging from 5 to 19 cm, and custom-made models may be ordered from some manufacturers. Stent length usually indicates the distance between the proximal and distal flaps of the stent, but in some models, stent length represents the length of the complete stent. The length of an endoprosthesis is generally selected to allow the shortest length possible while

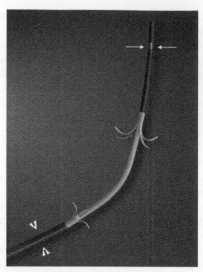

Fig. 2. Typical 10F design. Inner guiding catheter (*arrows*), stent (*blue*), and pusher tube (*arrowheads*) are seen. The stent is curved and contours to the duct and duodenum. (*From* Baron TH, Ponsky JL. Plastic pancreatic and biliary stents: concepts and insertion techniques. In: Baron TH, editor. ERCP. Elsevier; 2008. p. 153–63; with permission.)

simultaneously ensuring adequate drainage. Stents are usually inserted with their extremities protruding 1 to 2 cm above the proximal end of the biliary obstruction and 1 cm in the duodenum. A longer intraduodenal portion of the stent increases the risk of duodenal perforation.[18] A technique that can be used to shorten plastic stents that extend too far into the duodenum involved snare resection with the aid of the metal sheath of a mechanical lithotripter.[19]

MALIGNANT BILIARY STRICTURES
Distal Strictures (Not Involving the Hilum)

Nonhilar malignant biliary obstruction is mainly caused by periampullary tumors (including carcinoma of the papilla of Vater, cancer of the pancreatic head, and distal cholangiocarcinoma), more proximal subhilar biliary cholangiocarcinoma, gallbladder carcinoma, and (rarely) metastatic cancer.

Distal or mid–bile duct obstruction due to pancreatic carcinoma, gallbladder cancer, cholangiocarcinoma, and lymph node metastases are common causes of jaundice and often present with advanced disease, and a minority of patients with these conditions are candidates for surgery.

Several comparative trials have shown that self-expandable metal biliary stents provide superior patency and reduce the need for reintervention for stent occlusion compared with plastic stents in patients with malignant distal common bile duct obstruction. In a systemic review and meta-analyses, the median time to stent occlusion ranged from 111 to 273 days for metal stents versus 62 to 165 days for plastic stents. The median patient survival ranged from 99 to 175 days, suggesting that many patients die long before stent occlusion occurs.[1] No significant difference was seen between the metal and plastic stents in terms of technical success, therapeutic success, 30-day mortality, or complications. The prolonged patency of metal stents is offset by a substantially higher cost compared with plastic stents. Therefore,

predicting the prognosis of a patient before endoscopic retrograde cholangiopancreatography (ERCP) may allow selection of patients most likely to benefit. Two prospective studies in 213 patients concluded that tumor size and presence of liver
metastases were independent prognostic factors for shorter survival.[20,21]

Stent insertion in patients with malignant distal bile duct obstruction for temporary
preoperative drainage before pancreaticoduodenectomy is not uncommon because it
provides relief from jaundice while allowing assessment of operability. In addition, it
has long been proposed that reduction in serum bilirubin level may reduce postoperative complications. In this clinical situation, plastic stents are usually inserted rather
than metal stents because they usually remain in place for only a short duration and do
not interfere with subsequent surgical resection. However, preoperative biliary
drainage remains a subject of debate. A recent large prospective randomized
controlled trial comparing endoscopic preoperative biliary drainage using 10F plastic
stents with surgery performed 4 to 6 weeks later with surgery alone within 1 week of
diagnosis in patients with malignant distal biliary obstruction demonstrated that
preoperative biliary drainage increased the overall complication rate.[22] Both the
complication rate of the initial ERCPs as well as the need for reintervention were
high, and no improvement in postoperative complications was found when preoperative drainage was performed. Stent occlusion accounted for 15 of the 27 patients who
suffered cholangitis.

Hilar Strictures

Malignant hilar biliary obstruction can be caused by a heterogeneous group of tumors
that include primary bile duct cancer (the so-called Klatskin tumor), cancers that
directly extend into the bifurcation (eg, gallbladder cancer), and metastatic cancer.
Hilar cancers have a poor prognosis with less than 10% of patients surviving 5 years
after the diagnosis and most patients dying in the first year. Although surgery is the
only chance for cure, resectability rates are commonly less than 20%. For most
patients, palliation is therefore the goal of treatment.

The extent of duct involvement by perihilar tumors may be classified according to
Bismuth and Corlette (**Fig. 3**).[23] Type I tumors are completely below the confluence
of the left and right hepatic ducts; the right and left ductal systems communicate.
Type II tumors reach the confluence but do not involve the left or right segmental
hepatic ducts, and only the left and right hepatic ducts are separated. Type III tumors
occlude the common hepatic duct and either the right (IIIa) or left (IIIb) segmental
hepatic ducts. In type IV tumors, the hilum is obstructed with tumor extension into

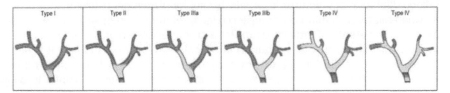

Fig. 3. Bismuth classification of hilar cholangiocarcinoma. Type I, tumors below the confluence of the left and right hepatic ducts (right and left ductal systems communicate); type II,
tumors reaching the confluence but not involving the left or right hepatic ducts (bile ducts
are separated); type III, tumors occluding the common hepatic duct and either the right (IIIa)
or left (IIIb) hepatic duct; type IV, multicentric tumors or tumors involving the confluence
and both hepatic ducts. (*From* De Palma GD. Malignant biliary obstruction. In: Baron TH,
editor. ERCP. Elsevier; 2008. p. 299–311; with permission.)

both left and right segmental bile ducts. Palliation with biliary drainage through endo-prostheses in patients with malignant hilar stenoses poses particular difficulties, especially in advanced lesions (type III and IV lesions). In these patients, the risk of incomplete drainage after contrast injection into the intrahepatic bile ducts leads to a high incidence of post-ERCP cholangitis. Retention of contrast and subsequent segmental cholangitis are risks associated with endoscopic attempts to treat advanced hilar lesions. The success rate of plastic stent insertion for hilar obstruction is lower than that of distal obstruction, although relief of symptoms with increase in quality of life can be achieved in nearly all patients successfully stented.[24]

In hilar tumors, self-expanding metallic stents (SEMS) have been demonstrated to be more cost-effective and require less subsequent interventions than plastic (poly-ethylene) stents.[25] However, the deployment of multiple SEMS can be significantly more challenging than that of multiple plastic stents.

In patients with strictures below the confluence of right and left hepatic ducts (Bismuth type I hilar strictures), jaundice can be easily palliated using a single biliary stent. For more advanced hilar tumors, it is important to realize that relief of jaundice generally requires drainage of about 50% of a healthy liver[26] or proportionally more in those with underlying dysfunction. Hence, unilateral drainage is usually adequate to relieve jaundice, and many studies have reported good results using a single stent in about 80% of patients with type II and III Bismuth tumors. No difference in efficacy has been shown between single stent placement in the left or right system. There remains a debate whether multiple hepatic duct drainage is necessary, but an increased risk of cholangitis has been described if only one side is drained.[27] In these more complex strictures (Bismuth type II to IV strictures), the unresolved question is whether adequate palliative relief of obstruction requires the placement of 2 (or sometimes even more) endoprostheses to drain each occluded segment or if 1 endoprosthesis placed in either system suffices. The necessity to drain all systems, if necessary combining endoscopic with percutaneous interventions, pertains more to the prevention of procedure-induced cholangitis caused by contrast injection in undrained biliary branches than to the effective palliation of jaundice. Generally, if both right and left lobes are imaged with contrast during cholangiography, bilateral stenting reduces the potential sequelae of cholangitis in contaminated but undrained areas. The use of pre-ERCP magnetic resonance imaging allows selection of segments or lobes to be drained, and therefore, contrast contamination into multiple segments can be avoided and more-effective palliation using unilateral stenting can be achieved.[26,28,29] Therefore, the decision whether to place a single biliary stent or multiple stents depends on the location of strictures, the volume of liver that can be drained to relieve jaundice, and the introduction of contrast into more than 1 segment.

Balloon dilatation of strictures is usually helpful for placement of hilar stents, particularly when bilateral stenting is attempted (**Fig. 4**). Moreover, in these strictures, there is still a role for stents of smaller diameter and the tapered pigtail stent design. For example, if bilateral stenting is required in patients with hilar obstruction, it is easier to place two 7F stents initially to gradually dilate the bile duct and then replace them later with 10F stents.[30] Tapered pigtail stents are sometimes helpful to allow passage across very tight strictures.

Management of SEMS occlusion

Another use of plastic stents is for the management of uncovered SEMS occlusion. Plastic stents can be inserted through the lumen of an occluded stent (in distal obstruction, **Fig. 5**) or stents (hilar obstruction). In some studies, this strategy is more cost-effective than insertion of uncovered SEMS.[31,32]

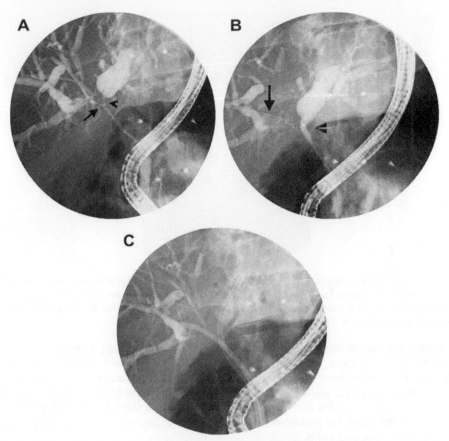

Fig. 4. Bilateral stent placement for hilar cholangiocarcinoma. (*A*) Malignant stricture involves left (*arrowhead*) and right hepatic (*arrow*) ducts. (*B*) Balloon dilation is performed of left hepatic duct stricture (*arrowhead*); note wire is in right intrahepatic duct (*arrow*). (*C*) Successful bilateral stent placement. (*From* Baron TH, Ponsky JL. Plastic pancreatic and biliary stents: concepts and insertion techniques. In: Baron TH, editor. ERCP. Elsevier; 2008. p. 153–63; with permission.)

COMPLICATIONS
Occlusion

The most important complication of plastic biliary stents is cholangitis or recurrent jaundice through stent clogging. Occlusion usually occurs within a few months after insertion, necessitating repeat endoscopic procedures for exchange of the clogged endoprosthesis. Much data have accrued about the process of stent clogging. Within a short time after stent insertion, proteins from the bile are absorbed by the stent material and may be used by bacterial cells as receptors for adhesion to the stent surface.[33] Bacterial glycocalyx formation provides a gellike biofilm of glycoproteins protecting the bacteria against destruction by antibiotics and the immune system[34] and also from the shearing effects of bile flow. Bacterial enzyme activity causes deconjugated bilirubin to precipitate, along with calcium salts of fatty lipids, forming a sludge, which ultimately blocks a plastic stent. More recently, scanning of occluded plastic stents has suggested that large dietary fibers due to duodenal reflux are a major factor contributing to the process of stent clogging.[35]

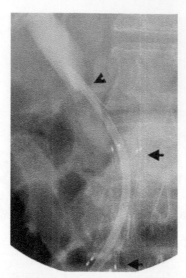

Fig. 5. Plastic biliary stent (*arrowhead*) passed through occluded metal biliary stent (*arrows*), which had been placed for palliation of pancreatic carcinoma. (*From* Baron TH, Ponsky JL. Plastic pancreatic and biliary stents: concepts and insertion techniques. In: Baron TH, editor. ERCP. Elsevier; 2008. p. 153–63; with permission.)

A clogged plastic stent is almost always easily removed with a snare or Dormia basket. In comparison, uncovered SEMS can only be removed within a very short period after deployment because the stent becomes embedded in the bile duct wall. Uncovered metal stent obstruction is mainly because of tumor ingrowth through the interstices of the stent or overgrowth of the ends of the stent. Metal stent occlusion is usually managed by placement of a plastic or a second self-expandable stent through the occluded stent.

Experimental animal studies have shown that plastic stents placed entirely within the bile duct (inside placement) have a longer patency than stents placed across the sphincter of Oddi.[36] However, clinical studies have not confirmed these results,[36] and inside placement increases the risk of stent migration.[37]

Migration

Stent migration, either proximally or distally, occurs during or after stent insertion in up to 10% of cases.[38] Stent migration may result in loss of stent drainage function and infection or perforation of the bile duct or duodenal wall. Endoscopic retrieval of proximally migrated stents is possible in 90% of patients,[39–42] although this may require surgical or percutaneous approaches. Techniques to remove migrated stents include snare or basket extraction, grasping with a rat-tooth forceps, inflation of a stone removal balloon alongside or above the stent and then withdrawing it, and passage of a guidewire inside the migrated stent followed by insertion of a balloon (retrieval or dilating) or specialized retrieval device (Soehendra screw extractor [Cook Medical Inc, Bloomington, IN, USA]) to withdraw the stent. If the stent has migrated above a stricture, balloon dilation of the stricture is usually required.

Breakage

A very rare complication is breakage of an endoprosthesis. In the past, polyurethane tubing was used; this material tends to harden with time and becomes brittle as described earlier. In the case of polyethylene stents, the only fragmented piece that has been described is the distal part, including the distal flap and side hole. This distal part is the most fragile part of the stent, which can break by repeated peristaltic movements. In case of breakage, the remaining part of the stent above the stricture can be difficult to remove.[40]

Complications Related to Stent Insertion

The risk of severe complications from endoscopic insertion is low at 1.8% (including a mortality rate of 0.6%) when preformed by experienced endoscopists. There is no significant difference in technical success, therapeutic success, 30-day mortality, or complication rates between plastic and metal stents. Biliary sphincterotomy is not necessary for inserting a single plastic biliary stent,[43] although one study suggested that sphincterotomy reduced the risk of pancreatitis when a single 10F stent was placed for hilar lesions.[44] Nevertheless, it is almost routinely performed during stent placement by some endoscopists because of the belief that it facilitates stent exchange during follow-up. Sphincterotomy facilitates the placement of more than 1 plastic biliary stent (eg, hilar obstruction) across the papilla.

SUMMARY

Plastic biliary endoprostheses have not changed much since their introduction more than 3 decades ago. Although their use has been challenged by the introduction of metal stents, plastic stents still remain commonly used. Much work has been done to improve the problem of stent obstruction but without substantial clinical success. Plastic stents are not costly, are accessible worldwide, can be easily inserted, and are removable.

REFERENCES

1. Moss AC, Morris E, Leyden J. Malignant distal biliary obstruction: a systematic review and meta-analysis of endoscopic and surgical bypass results. Cancer Treat Rev 2007;33(2):213–21.
2. Ferreira LE, Baron TH. Endoscopic stenting for palliation of malignant biliary obstruction. Expert Rev Med Devices 2010;7(5):681–91.
3. Soehendra N, Reynders-Frederix V. Palliative biliary duct drainage. A new method for endoscopic introduction of a new drain. Dtsch Med Wochenschr 1979;104(6):206–7 [in German].
4. Huibregtse K, Haverkamp HJ, Tytgat GN. Transpapillary positioning of a large 3.2 mm biliary endoprosthesis. Endoscopy 1981;13(5):217–9.
5. Huibregtse K, Tytgat GN. Palliative treatment of obstructive jaundice by transpapillary introduction of large bore bile duct endoprosthesis. Gut 1982;23(5):371–5.
6. Speer AG, Cotton PB, MacRae KD. Endoscopic management of malignant biliary obstruction: stents of 10 French gauge are preferable to stents of 8 French gauge. Gastrointest Endosc 1988;34(5):412–7.
7. Kadakia SC, Starnes E. Comparison of 10 French gauge stent with 11.5 French gauge stent in patients with biliary tract diseases. Gastrointest Endosc 1992; 38(4):454–9.
8. Matsuda Y, Shimakura K, Akamatsu T. Factors affecting the patency of stents in malignant biliary obstructive disease: univariate and multivariate analysis. Am J Gastroenterol 1991;86(7):843–9.
9. Pereira-Lima JC, Jakobs R, Maier M, et al. Endoscopicbiliary stenting for the palliation of pancreatic cancer: results, survival predictive factors, and comparison of

10-French with 11.5-French gauge stents. Am J Gastroenterol 1996;91(10): 2179–84.

10. Coene PP, Groen AK, Cheng J, et al. Clogging of biliary endoprostheses: a new perspective. Gut 1990;31(8):913–7.

11. van Berkel AM, Boland C, Redekop WK, et al. A prospective randomized trial of Teflon versus polyethylene stents for distal malignant biliary obstruction. Endoscopy 1998;30(8):681–6.

12. McAllister EW, Carey LC, Brady PG, et al. The role of polymeric surface smoothness of biliary stents in bacterial adherence, biofilm deposition, and stent occlusion. Gastrointest Endosc 1993;39(3):422–5.

13. Van Berkel AM, van Marle J, van Veen H, et al. A scanning electron microscopic study of biliary stent materials. Gastrointest Endosc 2000;51(1):19–22.

14. Seitz U, Vadeyar H, Soehendra N. Prolonged patency with a new-design Teflon biliary prosthesis. Endoscopy 1994;26(5):478–82.

15. Catalano MF, Geenen JE, Lehman GA, et al. "Tannenbaum" Teflon stents versus traditional polyethylene stents for treatment of malignant biliary stricture. Gastrointest Endosc 2002;55(3):354–8.

16. Raju GS, Sud R, Elfert AA, et al. Biliary drainage by using stents without a central lumen: a pilot study. Gastrointest Endosc 2006;63(2):317–20.

17. Reddy DN, Banerjee R, Choung OW. Antireflux biliary stents: are they the solution to stent occlusions? Curr Gastroenterol Rep 2006;8(2):156–60.

18. Saranga Bharathi R, Rao P, Ghosh K. Iatrogenic duodenal perforations caused by endoscopic biliary stenting and stent migration: an update. Endoscopy 2006; 38(12):1271–4.

19. Mutignani M, Dokas S, Perri V, et al. Post-insertion tailoring of plastic biliary stents: a novel technique. Endoscopy 2006;38(8):856.

20. Kaassis M, Boyer J, Dumas R, et al. Plastic or metal stents for malignant stricture of the common bile duct? Results of a randomized prospective study. Gastrointest Endosc 2003;57(2):178–82.

21. Prat F, Chapat O, Ducot B, et al. Predictive factors for survival of patients with inoperable malignant distal biliary strictures: a practical management guideline. Gut 1998;42(1):76–80.

22. van der Gaag NA, Rauws EA, van Eijck CH, et al. Preoperative biliary drainage for cancer of the head of the pancreas. N Engl J Med 2010;362(2):129–37.

23. Bismuth H, Corlette MB. Intrahepatic cholangioenteric anastomosis in carcinoma of the hilus of the liver. Surg Gynecol Obstet 1975;140(2):170–8.

24. De Palma GD, Masone S, Rega M, et al. Endoscopic approach to malignant strictures at the hepatic hilum. World J Gastroenterol 2007;13:4042.

25. Perdue DG, Freeman ML, DiSario JA, et al, ERCP Outcome Study ERCOST Group. Plastic versus self-expanding metallic stents for malignant hilar biliary obstruction: a prospective multicenter observational cohort study. J Clin Gastroenterol 2008;42(9):1040–6.

26. Vienne A, Hobeika E, Gouya H, et al. Prediction of drainage effectiveness during endoscopic stenting of malignant hilar strictures: the role of liver volume assessment. Gastrointest Endosc 2010;72(4):728–35.

27. Chang WH, Kortan P, Haber GB. Outcome in patients with bifurcation tumors who undergo unilateral versus bilateral hepatic duct drainage. Gastrointest Endosc 1998;47(5):354–62.

28. De Palma GD, Galloro G, Siciliano S, et al. Unilateral versus bilateral endoscopic hepatic duct drainage in patients with malignant hilar biliary obstruction: results

of a prospective, randomized, and controlled study. Gastrointest Endosc 2001; 53(6):547–53.

29. Hintze RE, Abou-Rebyeh H, Adler A, et al. Magnetic resonance cholangiopancreatography-guided unilateral endoscopic stent placement for Klatskin tumors. Gastrointest Endosc 2001;53(1):40–6.

30. Todd HB, RIchard Kozarek, Carr-Locke DL. ERCP. Philadelphia: Saunders Elsevier; 2008. p. 155–68. Chapter 16.

31. Katsinelos P, Beltsis A, Chatzimavroudis G, et al. Endoscopic management of occluded biliary uncovered metal stents: a multicenter experience. World J Gastroenterol 2011;17(1):98–104.

32. Yoon WJ, Ryu JK, Lee JW, et al. Endoscopic management of occluded metal biliary stents: metal versus 10F plastic stents. World J Gastroenterol 2010; 16(42):5347–52.

33. Yu JL, Andersson R, Ljungh A. Protein adsorption and bacterial adhesion to biliary stent materials. J Surg Res 1996;62(1):69–73.

34. Smit JM, Out MM, Groen AK, et al. A placebo-controlled study on the efficacy of aspirin and doxycycline in preventing clogging of biliary endoprostheses. Gastrointest Endosc 1989;35(6):485–9.

35. van Berkel AM, van Marle J, Groen AK, et al. Mechanisms of biliary stent clogging: confocal laser scanning and scanning electron microscopy. Endoscopy 2005;37(8):729–34.

36. Liu Q, Khay G, Cotton PB. Feasibility of stent placement above the sphincter of Oddi ("inside-stent") for patients with malignant biliary obstruction. Endoscopy 1998;30(8):687–90.

37. Pedersen FM, Lassen AT, Schaffalitzky de Muckadell OB. Randomized trial of stent placed above and across the sphincter of Oddi in malignant bile duct obstruction. Gastrointest Endosc 1998;48(6):574–9.

38. Johanson JF, Schmalz MJ, Geenen JE. Incidence and risk factors for biliary and pancreatic stent migration. Gastrointest Endosc 1992;38(3):341–6.

39. Chaurasia OP, Rauws EA, Fockens P, et al. Endoscopic techniques for retrieval of proximally migrated biliary stents: the Amsterdam experience. Gastrointest Endosc 1999;50(6):780–5.

40. Lahoti S, Catalano MF, Geenen JE, et al. Endoscopic retrieval of proximally migrated biliary and pancreatic stents: experience of a large referral center. Gastrointest Endosc 1998;47(6):486–91.

41. Sakai Y, Tsuyuguchi T, Ishihara T, et al. Cholangiopancreatography troubleshooting: the usefulness of endoscopic retrieval of migrated biliary and pancreatic stents. Hepatobiliary Pancreat Dis Int 2009;8(6):632–7.

42. Tarnasky PR, Cotton PB, Baillie J, et al. Proximal migration of biliary stents: attempted endoscopic retrieval in forty-one patients. Gastrointest Endosc 1995; 42(6):513–20.

43. Giorgio PD, Luca LD. Comparison of treatment outcomes between biliary plastic stent placements with and without endoscopic sphincterotomy for inoperable malignant common bile duct obstruction. World J Gastroenterol 2004;10(8): 1212–4.

44. Tarnasky PR, Cunningham JT, Hawes RH, et al. Transpapillary stenting of proximal biliary strictures: does biliary sphincterotomy reduce the risk of postprocedure pancreatitis? Gastrointest Endosc 1997;45(1):46–51.

Expandable Metal Stents for Benign Biliary Disease

Mihir R. Bakhru, MD, MSc[a], Michel Kahaleh, MD[a,b],*

KEYWORDS

- Metal stents • Self-expanding metal stent
- Benign biliary stricture

Benign biliary diseases include biliary strictures, leaks, and biliary stones. Benign biliary strictures (BBS) include postoperative injury, anastomotic strictures, chronic pancreatitis, primary sclerosing cholangitis, gallstone-related stricture, and other less common inflammatory conditions.[1,2] Postoperative strictures are most frequent, and include postcholecystectomy and liver transplantation–associated anastomotic stricture.[3] Chronic pancreatitis is a common cause of BBS, which can be difficult to manage endoscopically.[4–6] The clinical presentation of benign biliary diseases can be broad, ranging from subclinical (mild abnormalities in liver function tests) to complete biliary obstruction manifesting with jaundice, cholangitis, and ultimately biliary cirrhosis. The location of biliary strictures can be categorized using a classification proposed by Bismuth. Bismuth I strictures are located more than 2 cm distal to the confluence of the left and right hepatic ducts. Type II lesions are located less than 2 cm from the hepatic bifurcation. Bismuth III strictures are present at the bifurcation, whereas Type IV involves the right or left hepatic ducts, and Type V extends into these ducts more proximally.[2,7]

Before considering treatment, diagnostic evaluation is of utmost importance because malignancy needs to be excluded. Cross-sectional imaging with high-resolution computed tomography and magnetic resonance cholangiopancreatography allow for better visualization of the biliary tree than most other modalities.[8] In addition, these imaging modalities provide valuable information of surrounding structures, hence the stricture itself can be better classified before therapeutic endeavors are undertaken. Endoscopic retrograde cholangiopancreatography (ERCP) is often performed to obtain tissues sample, though is not always very accurate.[9,10] More recently, adjunctive diagnostic tools such as endoscopic ultrasonography combined

a Division of Gastroenterology and Hepatology, University of Virginia, PO Box 800708, Charlottesville, VA 22908, USA
b Pancreatico-Biliary Services, Division of Gastroenterology and Hepatology, University of Virginia Health System, MSB 2153, PO Box 800708, Charlottesville, VA 22908-0708, USA
* Corresponding author. Division of Gastroenterology and Hepatology, University of Virginia, PO Box 800708, Charlottesville, VA 22908.
E-mail address: mkahaleh@gmail.com

Gastrointest Endoscopy Clin N Am 21 (2011) 447–462
doi:10.1016/j.giec.2011.04.007
1052-5157/11/$ – see front matter © 2011 Elsevier Inc. All rights reserved.

giendo.theclinics.com

with fine-needle aspiration, intraductal ultrasonography, and even cholangioscopy have allowed further characterization and visualization with the goal of improving diagnostic capability.[11]

Biliary leaks can occur after biliary tract surgery and most commonly after cholecystectomy.[12] Postcholecystectomy leaks are usually from the cystic duct or duct of Luschka. Biliary leaks can become more complex when surgery is performed in the setting of severe cholecystitis or significant fibrosis, making cholecystectomy more difficult and prone to complications.[13] Endoscopic placement of biliary stents has become the first step in the management of postoperative biliary leaks. The number of and type of stents used, however, remains controversial.[14,15]

Choledocholithiasis can be cleared during ERCP, with success rates of up to 95%.[16–18] However, stone clearance can be incomplete, and temporizing measures such as stent placement can offer continued biliary drainage until repeat procedures and advanced extraction techniques such as mechanical and intraductal lithotripsy are used. In those patients who are at high risk for surgery or too ill, endoprosthesis placement can reduce the risk of biliary obstruction with resultant jaundice and cholangitis.[18]

TREATMENT OPTIONS

Therapeutic options for the treatment of symptomatic, benign biliary strictures include surgical, percutaneous, and endoscopic interventions. Surgery has historically been the gold standard.[19–21] Location of the stricture determines the optimal surgical approach, such as choledochojejunostomy for distal common bile duct strictures and hepaticojejunostomy for more proximal strictures.[22] Although successful with low reintervention rates, surgical morbidity is not insignificant, and can be upwards of 25%.[23–25] Less invasive procedures such as percutaneous drainage and endoscopic decompression have gained popularity, as they do not preclude surgery and are optimal for poor surgical candidates.[24] A percutaneous transhepatic approach with balloon dilation and placement of catheters has a success rate of upwards of 60%, with most recurrent strictures occurring within 2 to 3 years.[1,26,27] Misra and colleagues[25] showed a success rate of 58.8% with a follow-up of 76 months.

The endoscopic approach to benign biliary strictures has evolved over time to become an alternative to surgery.[28–30] Endoscopic therapy typically includes balloon dilation and endoprosthesis placement.[28,31] Several studies have addressed the effectiveness of plastic stents for treatment of benign biliary strictures.[32,33] The use of plastic stents typically requires placement of multiple stents with frequent endoscopic sessions, given the short duration in patency.[6,23,34–36] The current trend for the endoscopic treatment of BBS includes placement of multiple plastic stents with exchange every 3 months to avoid obstruction.[6,29,37–39]

Therapeutic options for biliary leaks focus on relieving transpapillary high-pressure gradient, causing bile to flow distally into the duodenum and away from the leak site.[40] This goal can be achieved endoscopically using stent placement with or without biliary sphincterotomy, which is quite successful for simple leaks but less so with complex leaks.[15] Incomplete extraction of bile duct stones can be managed with biliary stent placement using conventional plastic (straight or double pigtail), which allows for adequate biliary drainage. The objective is not only to provide a bridge to further endoscopic attempts or elective surgery, but also to potentially reduce the stone burden by facilitating fragmentation.[18,41]

Self-expandable metal stents (SEMS) were initially developed for palliation of malignant biliary strictures because their larger diameter results in an increase in duration of stent patency. More recently they have been used to treat a variety of benign biliary disorders.

UNCOVERED SEMS

Uncovered SEMS have been proved to allow sustained biliary drainage of malignant biliary strictures.[42] The limitations of plastic stents in patients with benign biliary strictures includes suboptimal stricture resolution as well as the need for frequent procedures to exchange stents to prevent recurrent cholangitis. Uncovered SEMS were the first available SEMS and thus the first to be used for benign disease. In one of the earliest studies, Foerster and colleagues[43] endoscopically placed uncovered SEMS (Wallstent; Boston Scientific, Natick, MA, USA) in 7 patients with benign bile duct stenosis (n = 6) or bilioduodenal fistula (n = 1) who failed dilation and plastic stent placement. There were no stent occlusions after a short mean follow-up of 8 months. An important study[44] gave insights to the tissue response of metal stents in benign disease. Choledochoscopic examination at 1 year showed complete epithelialization of the metal stent in all subjects. Median patency was 35 months (range 7–72 months), with 9 symptomatic stent occlusions occurring in 5 of 8 patients (62.5%).

There have been several studies on the use of uncovered SEMS in patients with BBS related to chronic pancreatitis.[45–48] Deviere and colleagues[45] placed uncovered SEMS in patients (n = 20) with chronic pancreatitis, and initially demonstrated relief of cholestasis for up to 33 months for 18 patients. However, repeat ERCP demonstrated that the stent was embedded within the bile duct and covered with tissue within 3 months. Similar studies confirmed these findings and the development of recurrent obstruction.[46,48] **Table 1** summarizes these studies.

PARTIALLY COVERED SEMS

In an effort to prolong the duration of patency in patients with malignant biliary obstruction, partially covered self-expanding metal stents (PCSEMS) were introduced. PCSEMS were found to be removable when placed across the papilla, offering the option of temporary placement.[49–54] Cantu and colleagues[53] placed PCSEMS (Wallstent; Boston Scientific) in 14 patients with common duct strictures due to chronic pancreatitis who failed prior plastic stent therapy. Strictures initially responded in all patients, but at a median follow-up of 22 months (range 12–33 months) 7 patients developed stent dysfunction, requiring reintervention. Of note, stent patency decreased over time, to 37.5% at 36 months, demonstrating that PCSEMS cannot remain in place long term.

The authors' group published a heterogeneous series of patients (N = 79) with BBS receiving PCSEMS (Wallstent) (**Fig. 1**). In 65 patients the stent remained in place for a median of 4 months (range 1–28 months) and were subsequently removed. Median follow-up after stent removal was 12 months (range 3–26 months). Three patients developed a stricture at the re-uncovered proximal portion, 3 failed primary therapy, and 2 developed duodenal obstruction preventing SEMS reinsertion, resulting in a success rate of 90% (59/65). Successful stricture resolution was noted to be lowest with strictures related to chronic pancreatitis (17/22, 77%). Stent migration occurred in 11 patients (14%), and 6 (8%) developed mucosal hyperplasia at the uncovered portion.[55] In a follow-up study, Sauer and colleagues[56] further analyzed long-term response in these patients after a mean follow-up of 910 ± 687 days. Sustained stricture resolution was seen in 59%. Of note, 15 stent migrations occurred and 7 patients developed tissue hyperplasia.

Table 1
Studies reporting endoscopic placement of uncovered metal stents

Study	No. of Patients	Etiology	Type of Stent	Median Stent Patency (Range)/Clinical Success	Median Follow-Up (Range)	Complications
Foerster et al[43]	7	Postoperative	Wallstent	8 mo/100%	8 mo	Sepsis/liver abscess (related to known bilioduodenal fistula) (1)
O'Brien et al[44]	8	Postoperative (5), (2), idiopathic (1)	Wallstent	35 mo (7–72 mo)/ unknown	64.5 mo (26–81 mo)	9 symptomatic stent occlusions in 5 patients
Deviere et al[45]	20	CP	Wallstent	33 mo/90%	33 mo	Symptomatic occlusion with tissue hyperplasia (2)
van Berkel et al[46]	13	CP	Wallstent	50 mo/69%	50 mo	Stent occlusion (3); migration (1)
Eickoff et al[47]	6	CP	Wallstent	20 mo/33%	58 mo (22–29 mo)	Stent occlusion (4)
Dumonceau et al[48]	6	Postoperative	Wallstent	17 mo/0%	17 mo	All stents occluded
Tringali et al[54]	18	CP	Wallstent	39 mo (5 mo–1.8 y)/44%	52 mo (26–121)	Stent occlusion (8)

Abbreviation: CP, chronic pancreatitis.

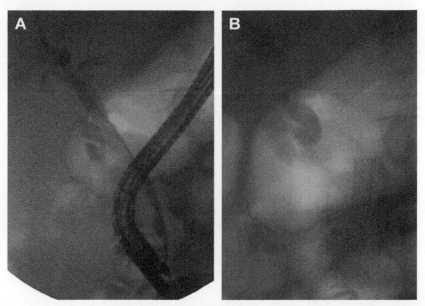

Fig. 1. (*A*) Fluoroscopic view of distal biliary stricture caused by chronic pancreatitis. (*B*) Fluoroscopic view after placement of partially covered metal stent. Note that the stent is placed below the cystic duct insertion.

Most recently, Chaput and colleagues[57] evaluated placement and removal of PCSEMS (Wallstent) in patients with anastomotic biliary strictures after liver transplantation. In this prospective, multicenter study of 22 patients, SEMS remained in place for 2 months, with subsequent removal in 20 (2 had distal migration). Temporary placement was not problematic, but the investigators did find extraction challenging. Complications with stent removal were minor and included self-limited hemorrhage and fever. Of interest, only those with migration or dislocation had persistent strictures after 3-month follow-up. Sustained stricture resolution was observed in only 45.6% of patients analyzed on an intent-to-treat basis. **Table 2** summarizes the studies using PCSEMS.

FULLY COVERED SEMS

Because of limitations related to partially covered SEMS, particularly epithelial hyperplasia at the uncovered portions, fully covered metal stents (FCSEMS) were introduced. Cahen and colleagues[58] published a series of 6 patients with strictures resulting from chronic pancreatitis treated with a 10-mm FCSEMS (Hanaro; M.I. Tech Co, Ltd, Seoul, South Korea). A 66% resolution rate was reported; however, 2 stents could not be removed and required plastic stents to be placed through the metal stent. More recently, the authors' group analyzed a FCSEMS with anchoring fins (Viabil; Conmed, Utica, NY, USA) to treat BBS of varying etiology. A total of 44 patients were included. Median time of FCSEMS placement was 3.3 months (interquartile range [IQR] 3.0–4.8 months), with resolution noted in 34 of 41 (83%) ($P = .01$) after median follow-up of 3.8 months (IQR 1.2–7.7 months) following removal. Complications were observed in 6 (14%) patients after placement, and 4 (9%) patients after removal, mainly pain and post-ERCP pancreatitis. A lower rate of resolution was seen with chronic pancreatitis (58%), and there was moderate difficulty in removing the

Table 2
Studies reporting endoscopic placement of partially covered metal stents

Study	No. of Patients	Etiology	Type of Stent	Median Stent Patency (Range)/Clinical Success	Median Follow-Up (Range)	Complications
Cantu et al[53]	14	CP	Wallstent	30 mo/37.5%	21 mo (12–33 mo)	Distal migration (2) Hyperplasia (5) Cholestasis (7) Cholangitis (5) Cholecystitis (2)
Tringali et al[54]	6	CP	Wallstent	20 mo (16–24 mo)/33%	35 mo (33–37 mo)	Stent occlusion (4)
Kahaleh et al[55]	79	CP, OLT, BDS, inflammatory, surgical	Wallstent	4 mo (1–28 mo)/90%	12 mo (3–26 mo) after removal	Migration (11) Stricture (6) Pain (2)
Sauer et al[56]	66	CP, OLT, BDS, inflammatory, surgical	Wallstent	198 d, 265 d/59%	909.8 d, 687.4 d	Migration (15) Hyperplasia (7)
Chaput et al[57]	22	Anastomotic strictures (OLT)	Wallstent	3 mo, 2.1 mo/45.6%	12 mo after removal	Minor pancreatitis (3) Pain (1) Cholangitis (1) Distal migration (2) Partial stent dislocation (5)

Abbreviations: BDS, bile duct stones; CP, chronic pancreatitis; OLT, orthotic liver transplantation.

138. Gaglio PJ, Buniak B, Leevy CB. Primary endoscopic retrograde cholecystoen-doprosthesis: a nonsurgical modality for symptomatic cholelithiasis in cirrhotic patients. Gastrointest Endosc 1996;44:339–42.
139. Conway JD, Russo MW, Shrestha R. Endoscopic stent insertion into the gall-bladder for symptomatic gallbladder disease in patients with end-stage liver disease. Gastrointest Endosc 2005;61:32–6.
140. Tamada K, Seki H, Sato K, et al. Efficacy of endoscopic retrograde cholecys-toendoprosthesis (ERCCE) for cholecystitis. Endoscopy 1991;23:2–3.
141. Hochberger J, Tex S, Maiss J, et al. Management of difficult common bile duct stones. Gastrointest Endosc Clin N Am 2003;13:623–34.
142. Bergman JJ, Rauws EA, Tijssen JG, et al. Biliary endoprostheses in elderly patients with endoscopically irretrievable common bile duct stones: report on 117 patients. Gastrointest Endosc 1995;42:195–201.
143. Chan AC, Ng EK, Chung SC, et al. Common bile duct stones become smaller after endoscopic biliary stenting. Endoscopy 1998;30:356–9.
144. Han J, Moon JH, Koo HC, et al. Effect of biliary stenting combined with urso-deoxycholic acid and terpene treatment on retained common bile duct stones in elderly patients: a multicenter study. Am J Gastroenterol 2009;104:2418–21.
145. Horiuchi A, Nakayama Y, Kajiyama M, et al. Biliary stenting in the management of large or multiple common bile duct stones. Gastrointest Endosc 2010;71: 1200–3.
146. Jain SK, Stein R, Bhuva M, et al. Pigtail stents: an alternative in the treatment of difficult bile duct stones. Gastrointest Endosc 2000;52:490–3.
147. Katsinelos P, Kountouras J, Paroutoglou G, et al. Combination of endoprosthe-ses and oral ursodeoxycholic acid or placebo in the treatment of difficult to extract common bile duct stones. Dig Liver Dis 2008;40:453–9.
148. Somerville KW, Ellis WR, Whitten BH, et al. Stones in the common bile duct: experience with medical dissolution therapy. Postgrad Med J 1985;61:313–6.
149. Pisello F, Geraci G, Li VF, et al. Permanent stenting in "unextractable" common bile duct stones in high risk patients. A prospective randomized study comparing two different stents. Langenbecks Arch Surg 2008;393:857–63.
150. Smits ME, Rauws EA, van Gulik TM, et al. Long-term results of endoscopic stent-ing and surgical drainage for biliary stricture due to chronic pancreatitis. Br J Surg 1996;83:764–8.
151. Bartoli E, Delcenserie R, Yzet T, et al. Endoscopic treatment of chronic pancre-atitis. Gastroenterol Clin Biol 2005;29:515–21.

stent, due to its anchoring fins. Ulceration and bleeding were seen after stent extraction (**Fig. 2**).[59]

A subsequent study of 55 patients with post–stent removal follow-up of 524 ± 298 days showed a success rate of 67% for those with chronic pancreatitis and 71% for other conditions. Given the modest resolution rates and significant complications, the authors do not recommend the use of FCSEMS with fins in the treatment of BBS.[56] In a multicenter retrospective study using FCSEMS with flared ends (Wallflex; Boston Scientific), 59 patients with BBS were treated. This stent has a distal loop (**Fig. 3**), which facilitates removal, and is the only metal stent approved by the Food and Drug Administration for repositioning and acute removal. Stricture resolution was demonstrated by imaging (16/18, 88.9%) laboratory (32/35, 91.4%), or symptom resolution (22/28, 78.5%). Choledochoscopy performed on 14 patients after stent removal confirmed stricture resolution in 12 patients (85.7%). Complications included abdominal pain (n = 7, 10.3%), pancreatitis (n = 3, 4.4%), and distal stent migration (n = 4, 5.9%).[60]

A newer stent using a nitinol covering (Niti-S, Taewoong, Korea) with unflared and flared ends was recently used in a cohort of 17 patients with common bile duct strictures secondary to chronic pancreatitis. The stent was removed after 6 months, with

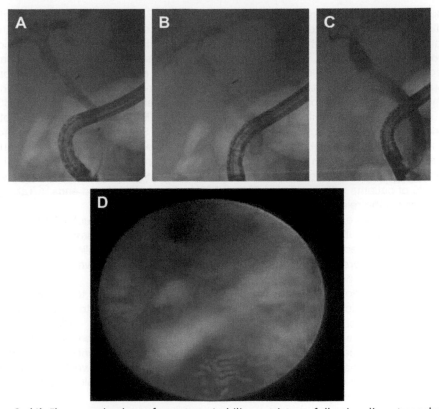

Fig. 2. (*A*) Fluoroscopic view of anastomotic biliary stricture following liver transplant (Patient B). (*B*) Fluoroscopic view of anastomotic biliary stricture after deployment of fully covered metal stent with antimigration fins. (*C*) Fluoroscopic view after stent removal showing ulcerated biliary epithelium. (*D*) Choledochoscopic view after stent removal showing ulcerated biliary epithelium.

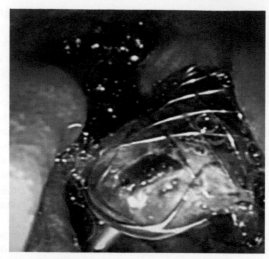

Fig. 3. Endoscopic view of a fully covered metal stent with retrieval loop.

follow-up of 3 years. Overall, migration occurred in 4 of 7 patients in whom stents with unflared SEMS were used, and 5 of 10 in whom flared ends were used. Of note, the group that had stents with flared ends placed had no intrabiliary migration, and stricture resolution was 87%. The group with placement of stents with unflared ends had resolution of 43%.[61] A recent multicenter, prospective comparative pilot study from South Korea compared two stents, both with flared ends at the distal portion, and either 4 anchoring flaps or flared ends at the proximal end. Of 43 patients with BBS, 22 received FCSEMS with proximal anchoring flaps (M.I. Tech) and 21 with both ends flared (Standard Sci Tech, Seoul, South Korea). Stents remained in place for a median of 6 months (IQR 4–6). No migrations were seen in the anchoring-fins group whereas a 33% migration was seen in the flared-ends group ($P = .004$). There was no difficulty in removing either stent type, and improvement of biliary stricture was noted in 91% of patients with anchoring fins and 88% of those with flared ends.[62] **Table 3** summarizes the relevant studies.

Overall, studies examining SEMS in the treatment of benign bile duct strictures have shown mixed results in stricture resolution. Earlier studies were small and showed success with a median follow up of only 2 to 3 years; few studies followed up beyond 3 to 4 years.[63] More recent studies with longer follow-up have shown similar stricture resolution and complication rates using different SEMS.[63,64]

With the evolution of SEMS design, research is being directed toward analyzing stent characteristics that lead to higher success rates. Factors to consider when choosing a particular SEMS include biomechanics, specifically radial (ability to expand) as well as axial force (ability of the stent to straighten). Isayama and colleagues[65] eloquently studied different types of covered metal stent characteristics, and determined that an ideal blend of both axial and radial force would provide the best clinical results. Studies are still under way to determine which stent has the best patency, fewest complications, and ease of removal.

METAL STENTS IN BILIARY LEAKS

Most simple leaks are successfully managed by endoscopic insertion of plastic stents.[15,21,66] In more difficult bile leaks, use of multiple large-bore plastic stents

Table 3
Studies reporting endoscopic placement of fully covered metal stents

Study	No. of Patients	Etiology	Type of Stent	Median Stent Patency (Range)/Clinical Success	Median Follow-Up (Range)	Complications
Cahen et al[58]	6	CP	Wallflex	3–6 mo (predefined interval)/66%	6 mo	Migration (2) Recurrent stricture (1) Difficult removal (2)
Mahajan et al[59]	44	CP, BDS, OLT, AIP, PSC	Viabil	3.3 mo (3–4.8 mo)/83%	3.8 mo (1.2–7.7 mo)	Pain (3) Post-ERCP pancreatitis (6) Migration (2) Occlusion (1) Stent unraveling (1)
Traina et al[73]	16	OLT	ComVi	6 mo/87.5% on removal	10 mo	Migration (6)
Sauer et al[56]	54	CP, OLT, BDS, inflammatory, surgical	Viabil	126 d, 74 d/67%	524.2 d, 297.7 d	Cholangitis (5) Migration (4)
Brijbassie et al[60]	71	Anastomotic stricture, BDS, CP, biliary leaks, undetermined, biliary adenoma	Wallflex	71.8 d, 42.6 d/91% by imaging and laboratory resolution	Not specified	Pain (7) Pancreatitis (3) Distal stent migration (4)
Tringali et al[61]	17	CP	Niti-S Unflared (7) Flared (10)	Predefined removal at 6 mo/43% (Unflared) 87% (Flared)	6 mo interval (up to 3 y)	Proximal migration with Unflared (4/7); Distal migration with Flared (5/10) Cholangitis—Unflared (3) Cholangitis—Flared (1)
Park, et al[62]	43	CP, BDS, OLT, postsurgical	FCMS with 4 anchoring fins (AF) (M.I. Tech, Seoul, South Korea); FCMS with both ends flared (Standard Sci Tech)	6 mo (IQR 4–6)/91% with AF; 88% with flared ends	6 mo (IQR 4–6)	7/21 migration with flared ends (6 distally)

Abbreviations: AIP, autoimmune pancreatitis; BDS, bile duct stones; CP, chronic pancreatitis; ERCP, endoscopic retrograde cholangiopancreatography; IQR, interquartile range; OLT, orthotic liver transplantation; PSC, primary sclerosing cholangitis.

with frequent exchange is required. Patients who have failed conventional endoscopic therapy using plastic stents or high-risk surgical candidates may benefit from SEMS placement, though limited data exist for such patients.[67] Those patients with challenging anatomy, such as Billroth II, may also benefit from SEMS placement due their ease of insertion. The authors' group analyzed 16 patients who failed to respond to plastic stent placement (n = 9) or had severe comorbidities (n = 7). PCSEMS (Wallstent) were placed, and remained in place for a median of 3 months (range, 1–17 months). The leak resolved completely in 15 of 16 patients and only one stent revision was needed, due to migration.[68] Wang and colleagues[69] used FCSEMS with anchoring fins (Viabil) in 13 patients with complex bile leaks, with

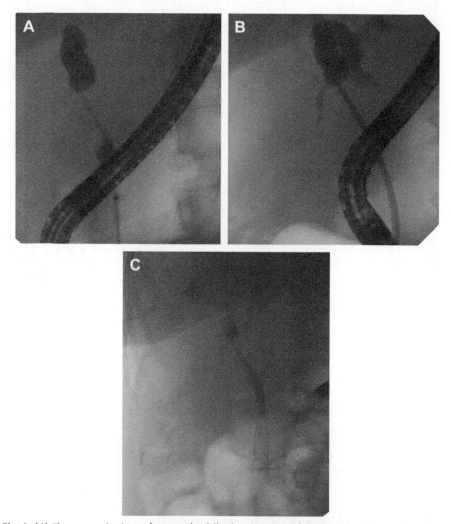

Fig. 4. (A) Fluoroscopic view of a complex bile duct injury with leak and stricture after chole-cystectomy. (B) Fluoroscopic view of the delivery system of a fully covered metal stent across the leak site. (C) Fluoroscopic view following deployment of stent with sealing of the leak and biliary decompression.

resolution in all. Complications included development of a stricture below the conflu-ence in 2 patients. In addition, 10 of 11 patients had evidence of biliary debris within the stent at the time of removal. There are limited published data on the use of FCSEMS with flared ends in the management of bile leaks, although initial cases re-ported so far have demonstrated good results (**Fig. 4**).[60]

SEMS IN THE MANAGEMENT OF CHOLEDOCHOLITHIASIS

In patients with complex biliary stones who have failed conventional endoscopic therapy and those thought to be too high-risk for surgery, endoscopic SEMS place-ment may offer a prolonged temporizing measure (**Fig. 5**) that allows for other methods of subsequent stone clearance, namely, extracorporeal shock-wave lithotripsy.[70] Minami and Fujita[71] used SEMS in the treatment of bile duct stones without sphincterotomy. In 38 patients an uncovered SEMS (Diamond; Boston Scientific) or PCSEMS (Wallstent) were placed to dilate the duodenal papilla and allow lithotripsy and stone removal. Successful clearance of bile duct stones was achieved in 36 patients (95%) with minimal complications; 2 stents migrated (one intrabiliary), one patient developing mild pancreatitis and one developing cholangitis. In a study by Cerefice and colleagues,[72] 36 patients who had failed endoscopic stone extraction underwent PCSEMS (Wallstent) or FCSEMS (Viabil) placement with mean follow-up 36.2 to 57.1 weeks. Complete stone clearance with stent removal was performed in 29 patients, while 4 of the remaining 6 required repeat SEMS placement to achieve ductal clearance. Complications included guide-wire perforation prior to stent place-ment (n = 1) and stent migration (n = 4, all Wallstents).

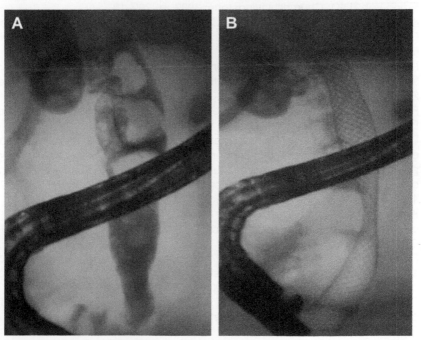

Fig. 5. (*A*) Large biliary stone burden. (*B*) Placement of a partially covered metal stent. Biliary stones are captured between the bile duct wall and stent.

SUMMARY

Although biliary stents have become an integral part of treating malignant biliary strictures, there is still a need for improvements to increase their long-term efficacy and to decrease their complication rates in the treatment of benign diseases. The ideal stent characteristics are yet to be determined. It is clear, however, that uncovered stents should not be used for benign disease because of their nonremovability and lack of long-term patency. Randomized, controlled trials comparing SEMS to plastic stents are required before recommending their routine use in benign conditions.

REFERENCES

1. Lillemoe KD, Melton GB, Cameron JL, et al. Postoperative bile duct strictures: management and outcome in the 1990s. Ann Surg 2000;232(3):430–41.
2. Judah JR, Draganov PV. Endoscopic therapy of benign biliary strictures. World J Gastroenterol 2007;13(26):3531–9.
3. Porayko MK, Kondo M, Steers JL. Liver transplantation: late complications of the biliary tract and their management. Semin Liver Dis 1995;15(2):139–55.
4. Deviere J, Devaere S, Baize M, et al. Endoscopic biliary drainage in chronic pancreatitis. Gastrointest Endosc 1990;36(2):96–100.
5. Smits ME, Rauws EA, van Gulik TM, et al. Long-term results of endoscopic stenting and surgical drainage for biliary stricture due to chronic pancreatitis. Br J Surg 1996;83(6):764–8.
6. Catalano MF, Linder JD, George S, et al. Treatment of symptomatic distal common bile duct stenosis secondary to chronic pancreatitis: comparison of single vs. multiple simultaneous stents. Gastrointest Endosc 2004;60(6):945–52.
7. Bismuth H. Postoperative strictures of the bile duct. In: Blumgart LH, editor. Edinburgh (UK): Churchill Livingstone; 1982. p. 209–18.
8. Kaltenthaler EC, Walters SJ, Chilcott J, et al. MRCP compared to diagnostic ERCP for diagnosis when biliary obstruction is suspected: a systematic review. BMC Med Imaging 2006;6:9.
9. NIH state-of-the-science statement on endoscopic retrograde cholangiopancreatography (ERCP) for diagnosis and therapy. NIH Consens State Sci Statements 2002;19(1):1–26.
10. Francois E, Deviere J. Endoscopic retrograde cholangiopancreatography. Endoscopy 2002;34(11):882–7.
11. Domagk D, Wessling J, Reimer P, et al. Endoscopic retrograde cholangiopancreatography, intraductal ultrasonography, and magnetic resonance cholangiopancreatography in bile duct strictures: a prospective comparison of imaging diagnostics with histopathological correlation. Am J Gastroenterol 2004;99(9): 1684–9.
12. Kaffes AJ, Hourigan L, De Luca N, et al. Impact of endoscopic intervention in 100 patients with suspected postcholecystectomy bile leak. Gastrointest Endosc 2005;61(2):269–75.
13. Spira RM, Nissan A, Zamir O, et al. Percutaneous transhepatic cholecystostomy and delayed laparoscopic cholecystectomy in critically ill patients with acute calculus cholecystitis. Am J Surg 2002;183(1):62–6.
14. Costamagna G, Shah SK, Tringali A. Current management of postoperative complications and benign biliary strictures. Gastrointest Endosc Clin N Am 2003;13(4):635–48, ix.
15. Mavroglannis C, Liatsos C, Papanikolaou IS, et al. Biliary stenting alone versus biliary stenting plus sphincterotomy for the treatment of post-laparoscopic

cholecystectomy biliary leaks: a prospective randomized study. Eur J Gastroenterol Hepatol 2006;18(4):405–9.

16. Cotton PB. Endoscopic management of bile duct stones; (apples and oranges). Gut 1984;25(6):587–97.

17. Vaira D, D'Anna L, Ainley C, et al. Endoscopic sphincterotomy in 1000 consecutive patients. Lancet 1989;2(8660):431–4.

18. Maxton DG, Tweedle DE, Martin DF. Retained common bile duct stones after endoscopic sphincterotomy: temporary and longterm treatment with biliary stenting. Gut 1995;36(3):446–9.

19. Hammel P, Couvelard A, O'Toole D, et al. Regression of liver fibrosis after biliary drainage in patients with chronic pancreatitis and stenosis of the common bile duct. N Engl J Med 2001;344(6):418–23.

20. Quintero GA, Patino JF. Surgical management of benign strictures of the biliary tract. World J Surg 2001;25(10):1245–50.

21. Sicklick JK, Camp MS, Lillemoe KD, et al. Surgical management of bile duct injuries sustained during laparoscopic cholecystectomy: perioperative results in 200 patients. Ann Surg 2005;241(5):786–92 [discussion: 793–5].

22. Nealon WH, Urrutia F. Long-term follow-up after bilioenteric anastomosis for benign bile duct stricture. Ann Surg 1996;223(6):639–45 [discussion: 645–8].

23. Berkelhammer C, Kortan P, Haber GB. Endoscopic biliary prostheses as treatment for benign postoperative bile duct strictures. Gastrointest Endosc 1989; 35(2):95–101.

24. Born P, Rosch T, Bruhl K, et al. Long-term results of endoscopic and percutaneous transhepatic treatment of benign biliary strictures. Endoscopy 1999; 31(9):725–31.

25. Misra S, Melton GB, Geschwind JF, et al. Percutaneous management of bile duct strictures and injuries associated with laparoscopic cholecystectomy: a decade of experience. J Am Coll Surg 2004;198(2):218–26.

26. Trerotola SO, Savader SJ, Lund GB, et al. Biliary tract complications following laparoscopic cholecystectomy: imaging and intervention. Radiology 1992; 184(1):195–200.

27. Pitt HA, Kaufman SL, Coleman J, et al. Benign postoperative biliary strictures. Operate or dilate? Ann Surg 1989;210(4):417–25 [discussion 426–7].

28. Geenen DJ, Geenen JE, Hogan WJ, et al. Endoscopic therapy for benign bile duct strictures. Gastrointest Endosc 1989;35(5):367–71.

29. Vitale GC, Reed DN Jr, Nguyen CT, et al. Endoscopic treatment of distal bile duct stricture from chronic pancreatitis. Surg Endosc 2000;14(3):227–31.

30. Davids PH, Tanka AK, Rauws EA, et al. Benign biliary strictures. Surgery or endoscopy? Ann Surg 1993;217(3):237–43.

31. Foutch PG, Sivak MV Jr. Therapeutic endoscopic balloon dilatation of the extrahepatic biliary ducts. Am J Gastroenterol 1985;80(7):575–80.

32. Huibregtse K, Katon RM, Tytgat GN. Endoscopic treatment of postoperative biliary strictures. Endoscopy 1986;18(4):133–7.

33. Smith MT, Sherman S, Lehman GA. Endoscopic management of benign strictures of the biliary tree. Endoscopy 1995;27(3):253–66.

34. Dumonceau JM, Deviere J, Delhaye M, et al. Plastic and metal stents for postoperative benign bile duct strictures: the best and the worst. Gastrointest Endosc 1998;47(1):8–17.

35. Draganov P, Hoffman B, Marsh W, et al. Long-term outcome in patients with benign biliary strictures treated endoscopically with multiple stents. Gastrointest Endosc 2002;55(6):680–6.

36. Costamagna G, Pandolfi M, Mutignani M, et al. Long-term results of endoscopic management of postoperative bile duct strictures with increasing numbers of stents. Gastrointest Endosc 2001;54(2):162–8.

37. Kiehne K, Folsch UR, Nitsche R. High complication rate of bile duct stents in patients with chronic alcoholic pancreatitis due to noncompliance. Endoscopy 2000;32(5):377–80.

38. Pasha SF, Harrison ME, Das A, et al. Endoscopic treatment of anastomotic biliary strictures after deceased donor liver transplantation: outcomes after maximal stent therapy. Gastrointest Endosc 2007;66(1):44–51.

39. Costamagna G, Tringali A, Mutignani M, et al. Endotherapy of postoperative biliary strictures with multiple stents: results after more than 10 years of follow-up. Gastrointest Endosc 2010;72(3):551–7.

40. Bjorkman DJ, Carr-Locke DL, Lichtenstein DR, et al. Postsurgical bile leaks: endoscopic obliteration of the transpapillary pressure gradient is enough. Am J Gastroenterol 1995;90(12):2128–33.

41. Katsinelos P, Galanis I, Pilpilidis I, et al. The effect of indwelling endoprosthesis on stone size or fragmentation after long-term treatment with biliary stenting for large stones. Surg Endosc 2003;17(10):1552–5.

42. Levy MJ, Baron TH, Gostout CJ, et al. Palliation of malignant extrahepatic biliary obstruction with plastic versus expandable metal stents: an evidence-based approach. Clin Gastroenterol Hepatol 2004;2(4):273–85.

43. Foerster EC, Hoepffner N, Domschke W. Bridging of benign choledochal stenoses by endoscopic retrograde implantation of mesh stents. Endoscopy 1991;23(3):133–5.

44. O'Brien SM, Hatfield AR, Craig PI, et al. A 5-year follow-up of self-expanding metal stents in the endoscopic management of patients with benign bile duct strictures. Eur J Gastroenterol Hepatol 1998;10(2):141–5.

45. Deviere J, Cremer M, Baize M, et al. Management of common bile duct stricture caused by chronic pancreatitis with metal mesh self expandable stents. Gut 1994;35(1):122–6.

46. van Berkel AM, Cahen DL, van Westerloo DJ, et al. Self-expanding metal stents in benign biliary strictures due to chronic pancreatitis. Endoscopy 2004;36(5): 381–4.

47. Eickhoff A, Jakobs R, Leonhardt A, et al. Self-expandable metal mesh stents for common bile duct stenosis in chronic pancreatitis: retrospective evaluation of long-term follow-up and clinical outcome pilot study. Z Gastroenterol 2003; 41(7):649–54.

48. Dumonceau JM, Nicaise N, Deviere J. The Ultraflex diamond stent for benign biliary obstruction. Gastrointest Endosc Clin N Am 1999;9(3):541–5.

49. Kahaleh M, Tokar J, Le T, et al. Removal of self-expandable metallic Wallstents. Gastrointest Endosc 2004;60(4):640–4.

50. Shin HP, Kim MH, Jung SW, et al. Endoscopic removal of biliary self-expandable metallic stents: a prospective study. Endoscopy 2006;38(12):1250–5.

51. Familiari P, Bulajic M, Mutignani M, et al. Endoscopic removal of malfunctioning biliary self-expandable metallic stents. Gastrointest Endosc 2005;62(6): 903–10.

52. Trentino P, Falasco G, d'Orta C, et al. Endoscopic removal of a metallic biliary stent: case report. Gastrointest Endosc 2004;59(2):321–3.

53. Cantu P, Hookey LC, Morales A, et al. The treatment of patients with symptomatic common bile duct stenosis secondary to chronic pancreatitis using partially covered metal stents: a pilot study. Endoscopy 2005;37(8):735–9.

54. Tringali A, Di Matteo F, Iacopini F, et al. Common bile duct strictures due to chronic pancreatitis managed by self-expandable metal stents (SEMS): results of a long-term follow-up study. Gastrointest Endosc 2005;61(5):AB220:T1314.

55. Kahaleh M, Behm B, Clarke BW, et al. Temporary placement of covered self-expandable metal stents in benign biliary strictures: a new paradigm? (with video). Gastrointest Endosc 2008;67(3):446–54.

56. Sauer BG, Regan KA, Srinivasan I, et al. Temporary placement of covered self-expandable metal stents (CSEMS) in benign biliary strictures (BBS): eight years of experience. Gastrointest Endosc 2010;71(5) AB110:347e.

57. Chaput U, Scatton O, Bichard P, et al. Temporary placement of partially covered self-expandable metal stents for anastomotic biliary strictures after liver transplantation: a prospective, multicenter study. Gastrointest Endosc 2010;72(6): 1167–74.

58. Cahen DL, Rauws EA, Gouma DJ, et al. Removable fully covered self-expandable metal stents in the treatment of common bile duct strictures due to chronic pancreatitis: a case series. Endoscopy 2008;40(8):697–700.

59. Mahajan A, Ho H, Sauer B, et al. Temporary placement of fully covered self-expandable metal stents in benign biliary strictures: midterm evaluation (with video). Gastrointest Endosc 2009;70(2):303–9.

60. Brijbassie A, Stevens PD, Sethi A, et al. Use of fully covered self expanding metal stents (FCSEMS) in the management of benign biliary diseases (BBD). Gastrointest Endosc 2010;71(5):AB298: T1519.

61. Tringali A, Familiari P, Mutignani M, et al. Self-expandable, removable, fully covered metal stents to dilate common bile duct strictures secondary to chronic pancreatitis: preliminary results. Gastrointest Endosc 2010;71(5):AB169: S1467.

62. Park D, Lee S, Lee T, et al. Anchoring flap versus flared end, fully covered self-expandable metal stents to prevent migration in patients with benign biliary strictures: a multicenter, prospective, comparative pilot study (with videos). Gastrointest Endosc 2011;73(1):64–70.

63. Siriwardana HP, Siriwardena AK. Systematic appraisal of the role of metallic endobiliary stents in the treatment of benign bile duct stricture. Ann Surg 2005; 242(1):10–9.

64. van Boeckel PG, Vleggaar FP, Siersema PD. Plastic or metal stents for benign extrahepatic biliary strictures: a systematic review. BMC Gastroenterol 2009;9:96.

65. Isayama H, Nakai Y, Togawa O, et al. Covered metallic stents in the management of malignant and benign pancreatobiliary strictures. J Hepatobiliary Pancreat Surg 2009;16(5):624–7.

66. Ryan ME, Geenen JE, Lehman GA, et al. Endoscopic intervention for biliary leaks after laparoscopic cholecystectomy: a multicenter review. Gastrointest Endosc 1998;47(3):261–6.

67. Baron TH, Poterucha JJ. Insertion and removal of covered expandable metal stents for closure of complex biliary leaks. Clin Gastroenterol Hepatol 2006; 4(3):381–6.

68. Kahaleh M, Sundaram V, Condron SL, et al. Temporary placement of covered self-expandable metallic stents in patients with biliary leak: midterm evaluation of a pilot study. Gastrointest Endosc 2007;66(1):52–9.

69. Wang AY, Ellen K, Berg CL, et al. Fully covered self-expandable metallic stents in the management of complex biliary leaks: preliminary data—a case series. Endoscopy 2009;41(9):781–6.

70. Maxton DG, Tweedle DE, Martin DF. Stenting for choledocholithiasis: temporizing or therapeutic? Am J Gastroenterol 1996;91(3):615–6.

71. Minami A, Fujita R. A new technique for removal of bile duct stones with an expandable metallic stent. Gastrointest Endosc 2003;57(7):945–8.
72. Cerefice M, Sauer B, Smith LA, et al. Covered self-expanding metal stents in complex biliary stone cases: long term experience. Gastrointest Endosc 2010; 71(5):AB299.
73. Traina M, Tarantino I, Barresi L, et al. Efficacy and safety of fully covered self-expandable metallic stents in biliary complications after liver transplantation: a preliminary study. Liver Transpl 2009;15(11):1493–8.

Self-Expandable Metal Stents for Malignant Distal Biliary Strictures

Jeffrey H. Lee, MD

KEYWORDS

• Self-expandable metal stents • Malignant • Biliary • Stricture

Obstructive jaundice can result from benign or malignant etiologies. This article focuses on malignant distal biliary obstruction and its management.

SHOULD DRAINAGE OF MALIGNANT DISTAL BILIARY OBSTRUCTION BE PERFORMED?

The most common cause of malignant distal biliary obstruction is pancreatic cancer and 70% to 90% of patients develop jaundice during the course of their disease. Pancreatic cancer is usually advanced at presentation, and curative resection is possible in less than 15% of patients.[1]

Biliary drainage before surgical resection is controversial; two investigators have reported it to be beneficial[2,3] but one has reported deleterious effects.[4] In patients with symptomatic malignant obstruction, biliary drainage relieves jaundice and improves symptoms, such as nausea, loss of appetite, and pruritus. In addition, if patients are scheduled to undergo chemotherapy, biliary drainage is essential to avoid the potential hepatotoxicity of chemotherapeutic agents. However, if a patient is asymptomatic and will undergo surgical resection within 1 to 2 weeks, drainage is usually not advisable. By refraining from trying to drain the bile duct in this setting, one can avoid unwanted complications, such as cholangitis, pancreatitis, and perforation that would delay surgery. However, when surgical intervention is planned for more than 3 weeks into the future or is not possible because of the advanced stage of malignancy and the patient is symptomatic, biliary drainage should be considered.

The author has nothing to disclose.
Department of Gastroenterology, Hepatology, and Nutrition, MD Anderson Cancer Center, 1515 Holcombe Boulevard, Unit 1466, Houston, TX 77030–4009, USA
E-mail address: jefflee@mdanderson.org

Gastrointest Endoscopy Clin N Am 21 (2011) 463–480
doi:10.1016/j.giec.2011.04.009
1052-5157/11/$ – see front matter © 2011 Elsevier Inc. All rights reserved.

giendo.theclinics.com

HOW SHOULD BILIARY OBSTRUCTION BE RELIEVED?

Malignant distal biliary obstruction can be managed by surgical bypass (choledocho-jejunostomy), by percutaneous transhepatic biliary drainage (PTBD), or by way of an endoscopic approach. Although biliary drainage was predominantly performed surgically before the 1980s, PTBD and then endoscopic drainage have since supplanted surgery for palliation of biliary obstruction. PTBD and surgical drainage are associated with considerable morbidity, patient discomfort, the need for repeated interventions, and occasionally death.[5–7]

Multiple randomized controlled,[7,8] prospective nonrandomized,[9] and retrospective studies[10] have compared surgical drainage with endoscopic drainage for malignant biliary obstruction and shown improved outcomes with the latter. A metaanalysis of 24 studies showed that endoscopic placement of plastic stents has the same technical and therapeutic success as surgical drainage procedures, similar quality of life and overall survival, a reduced risk of complications, and shorter hospital stay, albeit with an increased risk of recurrent biliary obstruction.[11] Plastic stents with their small lumen diameters are susceptible to loss of patency within an average of 3 to 4 months because of the formation of adherent bacterial biofilm and accumulation of biliary sludge.[12] However, self-expandable metal stents (SEMS), in their fully expanded state, have a lumen diameter three to four times that of plastic stents. The outcomes with SEMS have been shown to be superior to both surgical drainage and plastic stenting because of the increased SEMS patency from the larger lumens.[11,13–19] Today, endoscopic biliary drainage is the standard of care for the treatment of malignant biliary obstruction. PTBD is most often used when endoscopic retrograde cholangiopancreatography (ERCP) has failed. Surgical choledochojejunostomy is usually reserved for relief of dual obstructions of the bile duct and duodenum.

SEMS

Since the first description of the endoscopic placement of SEMS to relieve biliary strictures in patients in 1989,[20,21] the use of SEMS has been on the rise in the treatment of malignant distal biliary obstruction because of their relatively easy deployment and long duration of patency. By design, SEMS have a minimal surface area on which bacterial biofilm can form.[22] The median patency durations for SEMS have been reported to be 9 to 12 months when used for malignant distal obstruction.[16,17,23] In parallel with the advances in the design and material of SEMS, the application of SEMS has also expanded from their initial exclusive use for malignant strictures to their use to treat benign strictures. Many questions remain unanswered about SEMS. This article reviews the issues pertaining to SEMS in the setting of malignant distal biliary strictures.

The commonly used commercially available SEMS are listed in (**Figs. 1–5**) **Table 1**. The first widely used SEMS were made of stainless steel, whereas today most SEMS are made of the nickel alloy nitinol.

Recently, Weston and colleagues[24] reported a comparison of the clinical outcomes of nitinol and stainless steel uncovered metal stents for malignant distal biliary stricture. In this study, a total of 81 nitinol and 96 stainless steel stents were placed to relieve malignant biliary strictures. The most common cancer diagnosis was pancreatic (80.2% of nitinol stents and 62.5% of stainless steel stents; $P = .06$), and the most frequent site of stricture was the common bile duct (85.2% nitinol and 86.5% stainless steel; $P = .31$). Biliary decompression was achieved in 93.8% of the nitinol group and 86.4% of the stainless steel group ($P = .22$). Immediate stent manipulation was required in four patients in each group, and subsequent intervention for poor

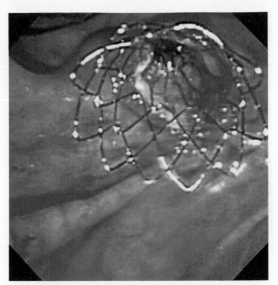

Fig. 1. Endoscopic view of deployed self-expandable metal stent exiting the papilla into the duodenum.

drainage was performed in 17 patients with nitinol stents (21%) and 26 patients with stainless steel stents (27%) at mean times of 142.1 days (range, 5–541 days; median, 77 days) and 148.1 days (range, 14–375 days; median, 158.5 days), respectively ($P = .17$). The overall duration of stent patency in the nitinol and stainless steel groups were similar (median, 129 and 137 days, respectively; $P = .61$), including in a subgroup analysis performed on patients with pancreatic cancer ($P = .60$) and common bile duct strictures ($P = .77$). Complication rates were low in both groups (early, 3.7% nitinol and 6.3% stainless steel; late, 2.5% nitinol and 3.1% stainless steel). Of note, 90% of patients underwent chemotherapy and 38% underwent radiation therapy in each group. At the present time, it seems there is no clear clinical advantage in one type of SEMS over the other.

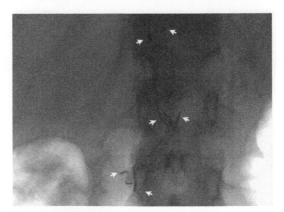

Fig. 2. Fluoroscopic view of nitinol expandable metal biliary stent across distal bile duct stricture. Stent ends (*top and bottom arrows*). Waist corresponding to stricture (*middle arrows*).

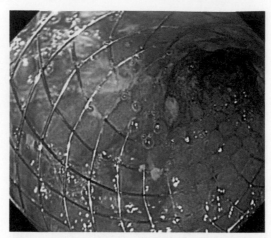

Fig. 3. Endoscopic view of self-expandable duodenal stent across a malignant duodenal stricture.

TECHNIQUES IN CANNULATING AND DEPLOYING SEMS IN MALIGNANT DISTAL BILIARY STRICTURE
Traditional ERCP and SEMS Deployment

The available imaging studies, such as computed tomography, magnetic resonance imaging, or magnetic resonance cholangiopancreatography, should be thoroughly reviewed. Particular attention should be paid to identifying biliary ductal dilation, foci of strictures, intrahepatic ductal involvement, volume of the liver affected, duodenal stricture, and gastric outlet obstruction. Because the biliary system is sterile until ERCP is performed, the benefits and risks of performing ERCP should be carefully assessed.

The bile duct is usually cannulated with a sphincterotome and a guidewire. Gentle, nontraumatic movements increase the odds of successful cannulation. Often, the mucosa in the setting of malignancy is quite friable and bleeds easily. Therefore, a traumatic approach can result in blurring of the anatomy from mucosal swelling and

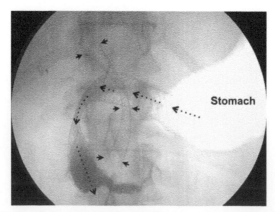

Fig. 4. Fluoroscopic view following combined enteral and biliary stent placement. Proximal and distal ends of the biliary stent (*solid arrows*). Lumen of the enteral stent from the stomach to the duodenum (*broken arrows*).

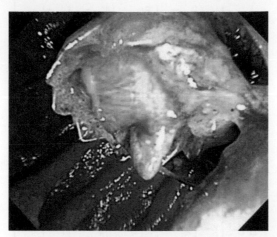

Fig. 5. Endoscopic view of occluded covered biliary stent. The distal stent lumen is filled with stone material.

bleeding, decreasing the chance of successful cannulation. Once biliary cannulation is successful, aspiration of bile should be done before injection to avoid dispersing bacteria that can cause sepsis. The minimal amount of contrast material needed to define the stricture and biliary anatomy should be used because of the difficulty of draining all the contrast material in cases of complex biliary strictures.

Once the stricture is identified, the length, location, and complexity of the stricture are assessed. The length of the stricture is often defined by using the sphincterotome under fluoroscopy. The proximal tip of the sphincterotome is placed at the proximal end of the stricture, and the sphincterotome is grasped at the biopsy port. The sphincterotome is then pulled back down to the ampulla under fluoroscopic visualization. Next, the distance of the sphincterotome that was pulled back from the biopsy port is measured and corresponds to the length of the stricture.

The predeployed metal stent is advanced over the guidewire into the bile duct. Most SEMS have radiopaque markers in their proximal and distal ends (some also have markers in the middle). For stents that foreshorten, the proximal marker should be placed well above the proximal end of the stricture. Once the stent is in the proper place, the outer sheath of the SEMS is slowly withdrawn by an assistant as the endoscopist is applying gentle pulling tension on the stent to compensate for the force of the stent propelling forward. Some stents can be reconstrained when partially deployed up to a certain point if the stent position is not optimal. Most stents that are reconstrainable have a mark on the stent beyond which the stent cannot be reconstrained.

Soon after a SEMS is deployed (see **Figs. 1** and **2**), flow of bile should occur. If a SEMS fails to expand and poor drainage is observed, balloon dilation of the stricture within the stent can be performed to facilitate immediate drainage. The size of the balloon should not be larger than the stent diameter.

Precut Needle-Knife Sphincterotomy

In many patients with pancreatic cancer, the regional anatomy is distorted because of the size of the tumor in the head of the pancreas or peritumoral inflammatory response. This distortion makes placement of the endoscope under the ampulla difficult. In this circumstance, achieving the proper angle for cannulation becomes difficult. One way to cannulate the bile duct is first to place a pancreatic ductal stent

Table 1
Specifications of various biliary SEMS

Stent	Manufacturer	Metal, Design, Coating	Covering Options	Length (mm)	Diameter (mm) Options	Radiopacity/No. Markers	Reconstrainability	Delivery Catheter (Fr)	Shortening (%)	Cell Size	Axial Force AF	Radial Force RF	Ends
Flexxus	ConMed	Nitinol	UC only	40, 60, 80, 100	8, 10	++ (tantalum)/4	No	7.5	<1	+++	++	++	Flared
[a]Niti-S	Taewoong Medical	Nitinol, hand-woven	FC, UC	40, 50, 60, 70, 80, 90, 100, 110, 120	8, 10	++/10	Yes (30%–40%)	8.5	No	++	+	++	Looped, flared
X-Suit NIR	Olympus Med	Nitinol	UC	40, 60, 80	8, 10	++/4	No	7.5	No	++	N/A	N/A	Rounded
Viabil	Gore Medical	Nitinol, laser cut, ePTFE	FC	40, 60, 80, 100	8, 10	++/2	No	10	No	N/A	+	++	Flared
WallFlex RX	Boston Scientific	Platinol, braided, silicone	UC, PC, FC	40, 60, 80, 100	8, 10	+++/4	Yes (80%)	7.5	40	+	+++	+	Looped, flared
Wallstent RX	Boston Scientific	Elgiloy, braided	UC, FC, PC	40, 60, 80, 100	8, 10	+++/4	Yes (80%)	7.5	40	+	+++	+	Open, flared
Zilver	Cook Medical Endoscopy	Nitinol	UC	40, 60, 80	6, 8, 10	++/4	No	7	No	+++	+	+	Flared

Abbreviations: ePTFE, polytetrafluoroethylene; FC, fully covered; N/A, not applicable; PC, partially covered; UC, uncovered.
[a] Widely available outside the United States.

and then to perform a precut needle-knife sphincterotomy upward from the pancreatic duct stent in the direction of the bile duct (11–12 o'clock). However, if the tumor extends down to the ampulla, a precut with a needle knife may not help because the bile duct is markedly strictured at the supraampullary segment. Furthermore, collateral vessels from portal vein thrombosis caused by the tumor may increase the risk of bleeding.

Endoscopic Ultrasound-Guided SEMS Placement

The role of endoscopic ultrasound (EUS) has been expanding from a diagnostic to an interventional one, and EUS is now increasingly used to guide biliary drainage. EUS-guided cannulation of the bile duct can facilitate obtaining biliary access when attempts at conventional ERCP-cannulation are not successful. There are three approaches to EUS-guided biliary drainage.

EUS-ERCP rendezvous technique

In this technique, using a 19- or 22-gauge needle, the obstructed bile duct is accessed under EUS guidance through the duodenum at a point proximal to the papilla. A guide-wire is passed through the needle into the bile duct and antegrade through the papilla. The echoendoscope is removed and a standard duodenoscope is inserted. The guidewire is then grasped by a forceps and conventional ERCP is performed.[25–36] Using this approach Kim and colleagues[37] reported that successful bile duct puncture and wire passage was achieved in 15 (100%) of 15 patients and successful drainage was completed in 12 (80%) of 15 patients. Although there were two complications, no bile leak or perforation was seen in this series.

In a variation on this technique, the left hepatic duct can be found by EUS with the scope placed in the stomach. The left hepatic duct is punctured with a 19-gauge needle under EUS guidance, and the guidewire is advanced down to the duodenum through the needle, stricture, and ampulla under fluoroscopic guidance. The echoendoscope is then replaced by a side-viewing endoscope, and the guidewire is grabbed and conventional ERCP can be performed.

EUS-guided transhepatic SEMS placement

Some have described placing SEMS over a guidewire through the stomach wall, liver, and then papilla. In this technique, once the fine needle is removed, the tract is dilated over the wire to 7 Fr or 8.5 Fr catheter using an ERCP catheter (Soehendra Biliary Dilation Catheter; Cook Medical, Winston-Salem, NC, USA). Subsequently, a SEMS is advanced over the guidewire through the therapeutic echoendoscope and deployed across the stricture via the papilla. Nguyen-Tang and colleagues[38] reported five successful placements of SEMS without any complications using this technique. The technique seems to be somewhat more invasive than others and requires expertise in therapeutic endoscopy. Clipping the gastric site of puncture should be considered to prevent leakage of gastric juice through the puncture site.

EUS-guided transluminal SEMS placement

In this technique, the bile duct is visualized by EUS and punctured with a 19- or 22-gauge needle under EUS guidance. The stylet of the needle is then removed and bile is aspirated. Next, a guidewire (0.018–0.025) is introduced into the needle and advanced further into the bile duct. The fine needle is removed, and after balloon dilation of the tract, a SEMS is placed over the guidewire through this tract.[39] The entry point of the bile duct should be near the ampulla and at least within the head of the pancreas (not at the common hepatic duct where bile leaks can occur). In a study involving eight patients who had covered SEMS placed using this technique the technical success rate was 100%, although one duodenal perforation occurred following stent migration.[40]

SPECIFIC ISSUES
Covered Versus Uncovered SEMS

Covered SEMS were introduced in the 1990s to improve the patency of SEMS by preventing tissue ingrowth, which occurs in up to 20% of patients who have SEMS placement.[41–43] However, unlike uncovered SEMS, which are integrated into the tumor or duct wall as a result of pressure necrosis, covered SEMS do not embed and have an increased risk of migration.[44] Although many retrospective studies comparing endoscopic placement of covered SEMS and uncovered SEMS for malignant biliary obstruction have shown prolongation of patency, with covered SEMS, prospective randomized trials have not shown a definitive advantage in one over the other (**Table 2**). However, covered SEMS were found to have a higher rate of stent migration.[42,43,45–49]

In a retrospective study of 77 patients who received metal stents (36 covered and 41 uncovered Wallstents; Boston Scientific, Natick, MA, USA) for unresectable distal malignant biliary obstruction, stent patency rates were not significantly different: 83%, 78%, 67%, and 54% at 100, 200, 300, and 400 days, respectively, in the covered stent group; and 83%, 66%, 54%, and 36% in the uncovered stent group. Stent occlusion occurred after a mean of 398 days in the covered stent group and 319 days in the uncovered stent group ($P>.05$). Stent migration occurred in three patients with the covered stent and one patients with the uncovered stent. Cholecystitis occurred in one patient with the covered stent but in none of the patients with the uncovered stent.[43] A more recent study comparing 278 patients with covered SEMS with 98 patients with uncovered SEMS for malignant biliary obstruction, however, showed a superior median patency rate (343 days) for covered SEMS over uncovered SEMS (184 days) ($P = .003$).[50] In a recent study evaluating the safety of placement of covered SEMS in 396 patients, stent migration occurred in 27 patients, cholecystitis in 13 patients, and pancreatitis in 4 patients.[51] Surprisingly, although stent migration rates have consistently been higher with covered SEMS in prospective nonrandomized and retrospective studies, no significant difference was noted in one randomized controlled trial.[42] The reported rates of acute cholecystitis with covered SEMS in various studies have ranged from 0% to 3.8%.[41,42] A recent study reported tumor involvement of the cystic duct origin as a significant prognostic factor in the development of cholecystitis in patients who received covered SEMS.[52]

Sphincterotomy Versus No Sphincterotomy

No prospective study evaluating the outcomes of endoscopic sphincterotomy (ES) for SEMS (covered or uncovered) insertion has been published, and there is no standardized practice for performing ES in patients undergoing transpapillary biliary SEMS placement. ES may secure easy access to the bile duct and facilitate therapeutic instrumentation of the bile duct. It also may reduce resistance to passage of the predeployed SEMS; improve immediate stent deployment or diameter at the level of the distal common bile duct; and enable a wider overall final stent diameter (which may result in better drainage, prolonged stent patency, and fewer reinterventions for recurrent jaundice). ES may also reduce pancreatitis by separating the pancreatic and biliary sphincters and preventing the SEMS from occluding the pancreatic duct orifice. However, ES is associated with a complication rate of approximately 10% (bleeding, pancreatitis, and perforation) and an overall mortality rate of 1%.[20,21,50,53,54] Furthermore, ES may prolong procedure time and costs.[55–58]

Banerjee and colleagues[59] reported one case of pancreatitis and five cases of bleeding in 27 patients who underwent ES just before SEMS placement as opposed no cases of pancreatitis (difference not significant) or bleeding ($P = .001$) in 77 patients who had biliary SEMS placement without ES. Stent migration was seen in 1 of 27 with ES and 3 of 77 without ES (difference not significant). Of note, 70 patients (67%) had uncovered SEMS placed and 34 patients (33%) had partially covered SEMS placed.

In the study reported by Artifon and colleagues,[8] 74 patients with unresectable distal bile duct obstruction were prospectively randomized to undergo biliary stenting with a covered SEMS with or without ES. Stent migrations occurred in six patients (16%) in the ES group and one (3%) in the group without ES ($P = .075$). No pancreatitis was seen in either group. Overall, complications occurred in 18 patients in the ES group (six stent migrations [16%], five mild bleeding incidents, four perforations, and three stent occlusions) and in four patients in the group without ES (three stent occlusions and one stent migration, 3%; $P = .006$). The authors concluded that placement of covered SEMS without prior ES in patients with distal common bile duct obstruction caused by pancreatic cancer is feasible and reduces complications.[8] However, one should keep in mind that in most patients presenting with bile duct stricture from a pancreatic cancer, the pancreatic duct is obstructed by the tumor and significant ductal and parenchymal damage and atrophy have already occurred. This condition perhaps contributes to the low incidence of pancreatitis in SEMS placement in malignant distal biliary stricture.

SEMS for Resectable Pancreatic Cancer

SEMS placement for biliary obstruction was avoided in patients with resectable pancreatic cancer for fear that the stent would interfere with subsequent pancreaticoduodenectomy. However, the approach at The University of Texas MD Anderson Cancer changed after the authors' favorable experience, which was published in 2005.[53] They found that in patients who underwent preoperative chemotherapy or radiation for locally advanced or borderline-resectable pancreatic cancer, placing SEMS before therapy was feasible and cost-effective.[53] In this patient population, SEMS placement reduced the number of ERCPs needed and the episodes of cholangitis that occurred during the neoadjuvant chemoradiation period. Furthermore, when biliary SEMS were placed and the proximal end of the stent was placed at least 2 cm distal to the bifurcation there were no stent-related complications during or after pancreaticoduodenectomy. Before this study, preoperative biliary stenting for resectable pancreaticobiliary cancers had typically been performed using plastic stents, with mixed reports of benefits versus complications.[3,60–62] A subsequent study comparing plastic stents with SEMS before pancreaticoduodenectomy in patients with resectable pancreatic cancer concluded that a short period of SEMS placement was more cost-effective than plastic stent placement.[63]

Obstruction of the Distal Bile Duct and Duodenum

A duodenal stricture complicates biliary stent placement in 10% to 20% of patients with distal biliary obstruction caused by pancreatic cancer. When stenting of both strictures is considered biliary stenting can be performed either preceding or following duodenal stent placement (see **Fig. 3**), and placement of both stents (see **Fig. 4**) in a single procedure may be an option.[64–66] In patients with symptoms caused by a significant duodenal stricture, the duodenal stricture may first need to be addressed.

Table 2
Comparative studies of covered SEMS versus uncovered SEMS

Authors	Year	Study Design	Number of Patients	SEMS Used	Patency	Complications
Isayama et al[42]	2004	Prospective	115 C: 57 U: 55	Ultraflex Diamond	C: 225 (11–1155) U: 193 (12–810)	C: Cholecystitis in 2[a] Pancreatitis in 5 (8.7%) U: Pancreatitis in 1 (1.8%) Hemorrhage in 2 (3.6%)
Yoon et al[43]	2006	Retrospective	77 C: 36 U: 41	Wallstent	C: 245 U: 202	C: Migration in 2 (5.5%) Cholecystitis in 1 (2.7%) U: Migration in 1 (2.4%)
Park et al[45]	2006	Retrospective	206 C: 98 U: 108	Wallstent	C: 148.9 U: 143.5	C: Pancreatitis in 6 (6.1%) Migration in 6 (6.1%) Cholecystitis in 5 (5.6%) U: Pancreatitis in 2 (1.8%) Cholecystitis in 1 (1%)
Gonzalez-Huix et al[84] (abstract)	2008	Retrospective	114 C: 61 U: 53	Wallstent	N/A N/A	C: Migration in 7 (11.5%) Cholecystitis in 2[a] Pancreatitis in 1 (1.6%) U: No complication
Cho et al[85] (Abstract)	2009	Retrospective	77 C: 39 U: 38	C: Wallstent U: Bonastent, Hanarostent	C: 227 U: 195	N/A N/A

Study	Year	Study type	N	Stent	Patency	Complications
Gwon et al[86]	2010	Prospective and retrospective[b]	116 C: 58 U: 58	C: Hercules U: Silver, Sentinol	C: [c] 98% 98% 91% 76% U: [c] 98% 83% 72% 57%	C: Migration in 2 (3.4%) Cholecystitis in 1 (1.7%) U: No complication
Kullman et al[87]	2010	Prospective	400 C: 200 U: 200	Nitinella	C: [c] 95% 83% 74% 50% U: [c] 97% 87% 78% 56%	C: Cholangitis in 8 (4%) Pancreatitis in 3 (1.5%) Cholecystitis in 2 (1.1%) U: Cholangitis in 12 (6%) Pancreatitis in 4 (2%) Cholecystitis in 2 (1.1%)
Krokidis et al[88]	2010	Prospective	60 C: 30 U: 30	C: Viabil U: Wallstent	C: 166 ± 87.7 U: 227.3 ± 139.7	C: Peritoneal irritation in 2 Biloma formation in 1 U: Peritoneal irritation in 3
Telford et al[89]	2010	Prospective	129 C: 68 U: 61	Wallstent	C: 205 (82–311) U: 159 (75–301)	C: Migration in 8 (12%) Cholecystitis in 3 (7%) U: Cholecystitis in 3 (7%) Pancreatitis in 1 (2%)

Abbreviations: C, covered SEMS; U, uncovered SEMS.

[a] Percentage for incidence of cholecystitis could not be calculated in the study because of prior cholecystectomies in some patients.

[b] Prospective for covered stents and retrospective for uncovered stents.

[c] Patency at 1, 3, 6, or 12 months.

A short duodenal stent can be placed without covering the ampulla, and once the stent expands, ERCP can be attempted by passing a side-viewing scope. Extreme caution should be observed not to dislodge the duodenal stent during ERCP. A series of 17 patients who underwent successful placement of duodenal and biliary stents was reported from MD Anderson Cancer Center.[67] Two (11%) of these patients had recurrent biliary obstruction from tumor ingrowth at 45 and 68 days, and two (11%) developed recurrent duodenal obstruction at 36 and 45 days after the initial stenting.[67]

During a combined procedure, removal of some of the wires of the duodenal stent mesh in the area of the ampulla with rat-tooth foreign-body forceps may enable bile duct cannulation.[68] Creating a window by removing some of the mesh wires of the duodenal stent using argon plasma coagulation is another alternative.[68,69]

Recently, duodenal stents with expandable lattices in the mid-portion have been used to facilitate identification of the ampulla and insertion of a biliary stent.[70] Moon and colleagues[70] reported a new duodenal uncovered SEMS (BONASTENT M-Duodenal; Standard Sci-Tech Inc, Seoul, South Korea) made of nitinol wire that has mesh with 2.5- to 2.75-mm cells and a 22-mm diameter. This duodenal stent is specifically designed for easy insertion of a biliary stent through the mesh wall of its central portion. The central 3 cm has a cross-wired but unfixed structure, as opposed to the fixed hook and cross-wired structure in the rest of the stent. The authors reported successful endoscopic placement of a biliary SEMS through the mesh of the duodenal stent in seven (87.5%) of eight patients. One mild case of pancreatitis was seen, but no stent-related late complications occurred.

COMPLICATIONS

Complications of SEMS include stent occlusion, stent migration, cholecystitis, and pancreatitis in addition to complications common to all endoscopic procedures, such as perforation, bleeding, and anesthesia-related problems.

When SEMS occlusion occurs (see **Fig. 5**), balloon sweeps are often performed to remove debris and sludge from the indwelling stent. In patients with an uncovered SEMS occluded by tissue ingrowth, placement of a second SEMS within the first stent is typically performed. A covered SEMS used in this setting seems to provide better patency than either a second uncovered SEMS or a plastic stent. In one study, the mean patency rates of second stent were 220 days for covered SEMS, 141 for uncovered SEMS, and 58 days for plastic stents.[71] Another study in patients with occluded SEMS evaluated the outcomes of placing a subsequent SEMS, placing a plastic stent, or performing percutaneous drainage. The median patency of the second SEMS (100 days) was significantly longer than that of a plastic stent (60 days) or percutaneous drainage (75 days; $P<.05$).[72]

Post-ERCP pancreatitis and cholecystitis are recognized complications of SEMS placement.[73,74] One study reported a higher incidence of post-ERCP pancreatitis with SEMS than plastic stents in patients undergoing SEMS placement for malignant obstruction.[75] However, the rates of post-ERCP pancreatitis in patients who received covered SEMS versus uncovered SEMS were similar. Conversely, other studies have reported increased incidences of post-ERCP pancreatitis and cholecystitis with covered SEMS than with uncovered SEMS.[42] The incidence of post-ERCP pancreatitis also seems to be higher in patients with an intact pancreatic duct than in patients with a dilated main pancreatic duct.[76]

If a SEMS is not placed in the desired position during the initial attempt, it can be grasped with a snare or a rat-tooth forceps and repositioned distally immediately after deployment (uncovered SEMS) or even later (covered SEMS). Some covered SEMS have a built-in loop at the distal end that can be pulled to collapse the stent, assisting with the desired manipulation.

When SEMS migration occurs, removal of covered SEMS is easier than removal of uncovered SEMS because tissue ingrowth often complicates the latter. In a series of endoscopic management of malfunctioning stents, removal was successful in 92% of patients with covered SEMS compared with 38% of patients with uncovered SEMS.[77] If an uncovered SEMS with tissue ingrowth is pulled forcefully, perforation of the bile duct may occur. Piecemeal removal of an uncovered SEMS using a hot biopsy forceps to fracture the stent lattice may be necessary.

Deployed stents are sometimes longer than expected and may impinge on the opposite duodenal wall. Such stents can be trimmed by cutting the metal lattice using argon plasma coagulation at a high setting.[78]

SEMS OF THE FUTURE

In patients with cancer, SEMS have served to alleviate biliary obstruction but typically have not provided any antitumor effect. A major limitation of SEMS use has been the substantial incidence of occlusion from tumor ingrowth and overgrowth and from tissue hyperplasia as a consequence of chronic irritation. To combat the occlusion problem and provide a therapeutic effect, drug-eluting stents (DES) have been developed. These were introduced first in the field of cardiology, and DES is now used as the primary stent for managing stenosis in coronary and peripheral arteries. In oncology, the theoretical benefit of DES would be to increase the drug concentration delivered to the tumor while minimizing the systemic toxic effects from chemotherapy, and reducing the risk of occlusion.

One antineoplastic agent that is a candidate for delivery by DES is paclitaxel, which has been shown in the laboratory to inhibit the proliferation of human gallbladder epithelial cells, fibroblasts, and pancreatic adenocarcinoma cells, suggesting that local delivery of this agent may reduce tumor cell proliferation in patients.[79–81] Lee and colleagues[82] endoscopically inserted paclitaxel-eluting metallic stents (Niti-S Mira-Cover stent; Tae-Woong Medical, Seoul, Korea) into the bile ducts of six mongrel dogs and control stents (covered Niti-S stent; Tae-Woong Medical) into five mongrel dogs. No technical complications occurred, and the authors reported that paclitaxel-eluting metallic stents are safe in normal canine biliary tracts. However, the incidence of mucosal hyperplasia was significantly increased in the paclitaxel-eluting metallic stents group.

In a multicenter pilot study, Suk and colleagues[83] placed metallic stents covered with a paclitaxel-incorporated membrane in 21 patients with malignant biliary obstruction. The mean patency of paclitaxel-incorporated membrane was 429 days (median, 270 days; range, 68–810 days), and the cumulative patency rate was 100%, 71%, and 36% at 3, 6, and 12 months, respectively. The mean survival of patients was 350 days (median, 281 days; range, 68–811 days). The serum paclitaxel level was highest between 1 and 10 days after paclitaxel-incorporated membrane insertion. Stent occlusion occurred in nine patients and was caused by bile sludge or clog (four patients), tumor overgrowth (three patients), or tumor ingrowth (two patients). Complications included obstructive jaundice in six patients, cholangitis in three patients, and stent migration with cholecystitis in one patient.

Although DES may ultimately enable delivery of local antitumor therapy and improve patency duration, the true benefits to patients may be limited by the fact that pancreatic cancer is a systemic disease with a high rate of recurrence, even after what seems to be a curative resection.

SUMMARY

SEMS have evolved from their relatively primitive form to highly sophisticated current models. There have been important developments in stent materials, designs, and technology. However, an ideal stent is still not in the hands of clinicians. An ideal stent would ensure efficient drainage; prevent occlusion by inhibiting tissue ingrowth; and provide effective antitumor treatment that confers a survival benefit (when used with a concurrent systemic therapy). However, given the ongoing research on stent technology, introduction of such a stent for managing malignant biliary obstruction may not be too far into the future.

REFERENCES

1. Rosewicz S, Wiedenmann B. Pancreatic carcinoma. Lancet 1997;349:485–9.
2. Klinkenbijl JH, Jeekel J, Schmitz PI, et al. Carcinoma of the pancreas and periampullary region: palliation versus cure. Br J Surg 1993;80:1575–8.
3. van der Gaag NA, Kloek JJ, de Castro SM, et al. Preoperative biliary drainage in patients with obstructive jaundice: history and current status. J Gastrointest Surg 2009;13:814–20.
4. van der Gaag NA, Rauws EA, van Eijck CH, et al. Preoperative biliary drainage for cancer of the head of the pancreas. N Engl J Med 2010;362:129–37.
5. Calvo MM, Bujanda L, Heras I, et al. The Rendezvous technique for the treatment of choledocholithiasis. Gastrointest Endosc 2001;54:511–3.
6. Lees WR, Heron CW. EUS-guided percutaneous pancreatography: experience in 75 patients. Radiology 1987;165:809–13.
7. Smith AC, Dowsett JF, Russell RC, et al. Randomized trial of endoscopic stenting versus surgical bypass in malignant low bile duct obstruction. Lancet 1994;344:1655–60.
8. Artifon EL, Sakai P, Cunha JE, et al. Surgery or endoscopy for palliation of biliary obstruction due to metastatic pancreatic cancer. Am J Gastroenterol 2006;101:2031–7.
9. Raikar GV, Melin MM, Ress A, et al. Cost-effective analysis of surgical palliation versus endoscopic stenting in the management of unresectable pancreatic cancer. Ann Surg Oncol 1996;3:470–5.
10. Maosheng D, Ohtsuka T, Ohuchida J, et al. Surgical bypass versus metallic stent for unresectable pancreatic cancer. J Hepatobiliary Pancreat Surg 2001;8:367–73.
11. Moss AC, Morris E, Leyden J, et al. Malignant distal biliary obstruction: a systematic review and meta-analysis of endoscopic and surgical bypass results. Cancer Treat Rev 2007;33:213–21.
12. Costamagna G, Pandolfi M. Endoscopic stenting for biliary and pancreatic malignancies. J Clin Gastroenterol 2004;38:59–67.
13. Davids PH, Groen AK, Rauws EA, et al. Randomized trial of self-expanding metal stents versus polyethylene stents for distal malignant biliary obstruction. Lancet 1992;340:1488–92.
14. Knyrim K, Wagner HJ, Pausch J, et al. A prospective, randomized, controlled trial of metal stents for malignant obstruction of the common bile duct. Endoscopy 1993;25:207–12.
15. Wagner HJ, Knyrim K, Vakil N, et al. Plastic endoprostheses versus metal stents in the palliative treatment of malignant hilar biliary obstruction: a prospective and randomized trial. Endoscopy 1993;25:213–8.

16. Prat F, Chapat O, Ducot B, et al. A randomized trial of endoscopic drainage methods for inoperable malignant strictures of the common bile duct. Gastrointest Endosc 1998;47:1–7.

17. Kaassis M, Boyer J, Dumas R, et al. Plastic or metal stents for malignant stricture of the common bile duct? Results of a randomized prospective study. Gastrointest Endosc 2003;57:178–82.

18. Moses PL, Alan BN, Gordon SR, et al. A randomized multicenter trial comparing plastic to covered metal stents for the palliation of lower malignant biliary obstruction [abstract]. Gastrointest Endosc 2006;63:AB289.

19. Soderlund C, Linder S. Covered metal versus plastic stents for malignant common bile duct stenosis: a prospective, randomized, controlled trial. Gastrointest Endosc 2006;63:986–95.

20. Neuhaus H, Hagenmuller F, Classen M. Self-expanding biliary stents: preliminary clinical experience. Endoscopy 1989;21:225–8.

21. Huibregtse K, Cheng J, Coene PP, et al. Endoscopic placement of expandable metal stents for biliary strictures: a preliminary report on experience with 33 patients. Endoscopy 1989;21:280–2.

22. Leung JW, Liu YL, Chan RC, et al. Effects of adherence factors and human bile on bacterial attachment and biliary stent blockage: an in vitro study. Gastrointest Endosc 2002;56:72–7.

23. Yeoh KG, Zimmerman MJ, Cunningham JT, et al. Comparative costs of metal versus plastic biliary stent strategies for malignant obstructive jaundice by decision analysis. Gastrointest Endosc 1999;49:466–71.

24. Weston BR, Ross WA, Liu J, et al. Clinical outcomes of nitinol and stainless steel uncovered metal stents for malignant biliary strictures: is there a difference. Gastrointest Endosc 2010;72(6):1195–200.

25. Mallery S, Matlock J, Freeman ML. EUS-guided rendezvous drainage of obstructed biliary and pancreatic ducts: report of 6 cases. Gastrointest Endosc 2004;59:100–17.

26. Kahaleh M, Yoshida C, Kane L, et al. Interventional EUS cholangiography: a report of five cases. Gastrointest Endosc 2004;60:138–42.

27. Püspök A, Lomoschitz F, Dejaco C, et al. Endoscopic ultrasound guided therapy of benign and malignant biliary obstruction: a case series. Am J Gastroenterol 2005;100:1743–7.

28. Wiersema MJ, Sandusky D, Carr R, et al. Endosonography-guided cholangiopancreatography. Gastrointest Endosc 1996;43:102–6.

29. Giovannini M, Moutardier V, Pesenti C, et al. Endoscopic ultrasound guided bilioduodenal anastomosis: a new technique for biliary drainage. Endoscopy 2001; 33:898–900.

30. Burmester E, Niehaus J, Leineweber T, et al. EUS-cholangiodrainage of the bile duct: report of 4 cases. Gastrointest Endosc 2003;57:246–50.

31. Giovannini M, Dotti M, Bories E, et al. Hepaticogastrostomy by echoendoscopy as a palliative treatment in a patient with metastatic biliary obstruction. Endoscopy 2003;35:1076–8.

32. Kahaleh M, Hernandez AJ, Tokar J, et al. Interventional EUS-guided cholangiography: evaluation of a technique in evolution. Gastrointest Endosc 2006;61:52–9.

33. Will U, Thieme A, Fueldner F, et al. Treatment of biliary obstruction in selected patients by endoscopic ultrasonography (EUS)-guided transluminal biliary drainage. Endoscopy 2007;39:292–5.

34. Bories E, Pesenti C, Caillol F, et al. Transgastric endoscopic ultrasonography-guided biliary drainage: result of a pilot study. Endoscopy 2007;39:287–91.

35. Gupta K, Mallery S, Hunter D, et al. Endoscopic ultrasound and percutaneous access for endoscopic biliary and pancreatic drainage after initially failed ERCP. Rev Gastroenterol Disord 2007;7:22–37.
36. Ponnudurai R, Giovannini M, Deviere J, et al. EUS guided hepatico gastrostomy [abstract]. Gastrointest Endosc 2004;58:AB4.
37. Kim YS, Gupta K, Mallery S, et al. Endoscopic ultrasound rendezvous for bile duct access using a transduodenal approach: cumulative experience at a single center. A case series. Endoscopy 2010;42:496–502.
38. Nguyen-Tang T, Binmoeller KF, Sanchez-Yague A, et al. Endoscopic ultrasound (EUS)-guided transhepatic anterograde self-expandable metal stent (SEMS) placement across malignant biliary obstruction. Endoscopy 2010;42:232–6.
39. Ito K, Fujita N, Noda Y, et al. Endosonography-guided biliary drainage with one-step placement of a newly developed fully covered metal stent followed by duodenal stenting for pancreatic head cancer. Diagn Ther Endosc 2010; 2010(426534):1–4.
40. Siddiqui AA, Sreenarasimhaiah J, Lara LF, et al. Endoscopic ultrasound-guided transduodenal placement of a fully covered metal stent for palliative biliary drainage in patients with malignant biliary obstruction. Surg Endosc 2011; 25(2):549–55.
41. Kahaleh M, Tokar J, Conaway MR, et al. Efficacy and complications of covered Wallstents in malignant distal biliary obstruction. Gastrointest Endosc 2005;61: 528–33.
42. Isayama H, Komatsu Y, Tsujino T, et al. A prospective randomised study of "covered" versus "uncovered" diamond stents for the management of distal malignant biliary obstruction. Gut 2004;53:729–34.
43. Yoon WJ, Lee JK, Lee KH, et al. A comparison of covered and uncovered Wallstents for the management of distal malignant biliary obstruction. Gastrointest Endosc 2006;63(7):996–1000.
44. Bethge N, Sommer A, Gross U, et al. Human tissue responses to metal stents implanted in vivo for the palliation of malignant stenoses. Gastrointest Endosc 1996; 43:596–602.
45. Park do H, Kim MH, Choi JS, et al. Covered versus uncovered wallstent for malignant extrahepatic biliary obstruction: a cohort comparative analysis. Clin Gastroenterol Hepatol 2006;4:790–6.
46. Miyayama S, Matsui O, Akakura Y, et al. Efficacy of covered metallic stents in the treatment of unresectable malignant biliary obstruction. Cardiovasc Intervent Radiol 2004;27:349–54.
47. Shim CS, Lee YH, Cho YD, et al. Preliminary results of a new covered biliary metal stent for malignant biliary obstruction. Endoscopy 1998;30:345–50.
48. Nakamura T, Hirai R, Kitagawa M, et al. Treatment of common bile duct obstruction by pancreatic cancer using various stents: single-center experience. Cardiovasc Intervent Radiol 2002;25:373–80.
49. Smits ME, Rauws EAJ, Groen AK, et al. Preliminary results of a prospective randomized study of partially covered wallstents vs noncovered wallstents. Gastrointest Endosc 1995;41:416.
50. Isayama H, Nakai Y, Togawa O, et al. Covered metallic stents in the management of malignant and benign pancreatobiliary strictures. J Hepatobiliary Pancreat Surg 2009;16:624–7.
51. Ho H, Mahajan A, Gosain S, et al. Management of complications associated with partially covered biliary metal stents. Dig Dis Sci 2010;55:516–22.

52. Suk KT, Kim HS, Kim JW, et al. Risk factors for cholecystitis after metal stent placement in malignant biliary obstruction. Gastrointest Endosc 2006;64:522–9.
53. Wasan SM, Ross WA, Staerkel GA, et al. Use of expandable metallic biliary stents in resectable pancreatic cancer. Am J Gastroenterol 2005;100:2056–61.
54. Arguedas MR, Heudebert GH, Stinnett AA, et al. Biliary stents in malignant obstructive jaundice due to pancreatic carcinoma: a cost-effectiveness analysis. Am J Gastroenterol 2002;97:898–904.
55. Giorgio PD, Luca LD. Comparison of treatment outcomes between biliary plastic stent placements with and without endoscopic sphincterotomy for inoperable malignant common bile duct obstruction. World J Gastroenterol 2004;10(8):1212–4.
56. Moss AC, Morris E, Mac Mathuna P. Palliative biliary stents for obstructing pancreatic carcinoma. Cochrane Database Syst Rev 2006;2:CD004200.
57. Freeman ML, Nelson DB, Sherman S, et al. Complication of endoscopic biliary sphincterotomy. N Engl J Med 1996;335:909–18.
58. Folkers MT, Disario JA, Adler DG. Long-term complications of endoscopic biliary sphincterotomy for choledocholithiasis: a North-American perspective. Am J Gastroenterol 2009;104(11):2868–9.
59. Banerjee N, Hilden K, Baron TH, et al. Endoscopic biliary sphincterotomy is not required for transpapillary SEMS placement for biliary obstruction. Dig Dis Sci 2011;56(2):591–5.
60. Wang Q, Gurusamy KS, Lin H, et al. Preoperative biliary drainage for obstructive jaundice. Cochrane Database Syst Rev 2008;3:CD005444.
61. Sewnath ME, Karsten TM, Prins MH, et al. A meta-analysis on the efficacy of preoperative biliary drainage for tumors causing obstructive jaundice. Ann Surg 2002;236:17–27.
62. Baron TH, Kozarek RA. Preoperative biliary stents in pancreatic cancer: proceed with caution. N Engl J Med 2010;362:170–2.
63. Chen VK, Arguedas MR, Baron TH. Expandable metal biliary stents before pancreaticoduodenectomy for pancreatic cancer: a Monte-Carlo decision analysis. Clin Gastroenterol Hepatol 2005;3:1229–37.
64. Freeman ML, Cass OW. Interlocking expandable metal stents for simultaneous treatment of malignant biliary and duodenal obstruction. Gastrointest Endosc 1996;44:98–9.
65. Maire F, Hammel P, Ponsot P, et al. Long-term outcome of biliary and duodenal stents in palliative treatment of patients with unresectable adenocarcinoma of the head of pancreas. Am J Gastroenterol 2006;101:735–42.
66. Profili S, Feo CF, Meloni GB, et al. Combined biliary and duodenal stenting for palliation of pancreatic cancer. Scand J Gastroenterol 2003;38:1099–102.
67. Kaw M, Singh S, Gagneja H. Clinical outcome of simultaneous self expandable metal stents for palliation of malignant biliary and duodenal obstruction. Surg Endosc 2003;17:457–61.
68. Mutignani M, Tringali A, Shah SG, et al. Combined endoscopic stent insertion in malignant biliary and duodenal obstruction. Endoscopy 2007;39:440–7.
69. Vanbiervliet G, Demarquay JF, Dumas R, et al. Endoscopic insertion of biliary stents in 18 patients with metallic duodenal stents who developed secondary malignant obstructive jaundice. Gastroenterol Clin Biol 2004;28:1209–13.
70. Moon JH, Choi HJ, Ko BM, et al. Combined endoscopic stent-in-stent placement for malignant biliary and duodenal obstruction by using a new duodenal metal stent (with videos). Gastrointest Endosc 2009;70:772–7.

71. Togawa O, Kawabe T, Isayama H, et al. Management of occluded uncovered metallic stents in patients with malignant distal biliary obstructions using covered metallic stents. J Clin Gastroenterol 2008;42:546–9.

72. Ridtitid W, Rerknimitr R, Janchai A, et al. Outcome of second interventions for occluded metallic stents in patients with malignant biliary obstruction. Surg Endosc 2010;24(9):2216–20.

73. Dolan R, Pinkas H, Brady PG. Acute cholecystitis after palliative stenting for malignant obstruction of the biliary tree. Gastrointest Endosc 1993;39:447–9.

74. Leung JW, Chung SC, Sung JY, et al. Acute cholecystitis after stenting of the common bile duct for obstruction secondary to pancreatic cancer. Gastrointest Endosc 1989;35:109–10.

75. Cote GA, Kumar N, Ansstas M, et al. Risk of post-ERCP pancreatitis with placement of self-expandable metallic stents. Gastrointest Endosc 2010;72:755–7.

76. Isayama H, Kawabe T, Nakai Y, et al. Cholecystitis after metallic stent placement in patients with malignant distal biliary obstruction. Clin Gastroenterol Hepatol 2006;4:1148–53.

77. Familiari P, Bulajic M, Mutignani M, et al. Endoscopic removal of malfunctioning biliary self-expandable metallic stents. Gastrointest Endosc 2005;62:903–10.

78. Vanbiervliet G, Piche T, Caroli-Bosc FX, et al. Endoscopic argon plasma trimming of biliary and gastrointestinal metallic stents. Endoscopy 2005;37:434–8.

79. Rowinsky EK, Donehover RC. Paclitaxel (Taxol). N Engl J Med 1995;332:1004–14.

80. Kalinowski M, Alfke H, Kleb B, et al. Paclitaxel inhibits proliferation of cell lines responsible for metal stent obstruction: possible topical application in malignant bile duct obstructions. Invest Radiol 2002;37:399–404.

81. Dhanikula AB, Panchagnula R. Localized paclitaxel delivery. Int J Pharm 1999; 183:85–100.

82. Lee SS, Shin JH, Han JM, et al. Histologic influence of paclitaxel-eluting covered metallic stents in a canine biliary model. Gastrointest Endosc 2009;69(6):1140–7.

83. Suk KT, Kim JW, Kim HS, et al. Human application of a metallic stent covered with a paclitaxel-incorporated membrane for malignant biliary obstruction: multicenter pilot study. Gastrointest Endosc 2007;66:798–803.

84. Gonzalez-Huix F, Huertas C, Figa M, et al. A randomized controlled trial comparing the covered (cSEMS) versus uncovered self-expandable metal stents (uSEMS) for the palliation of malignant distal biliary obstruction: interim analysis [abstract]. Gastrointest Endosc 2008;67:AB166.

85. Cho YD, Cheon YK, Yoo KS, et al. Uncovered versus covered self expanding metal stents for inoperable malignant distal biliary obstruction: a prospective randomized multicenter study [abstract]. Gastrointest Endosc 2009;69:AB137.

86. Gwon DI, Ko GY, Kim JH, et al. A comparative analysis of PTFE-covered and uncovered stents for palliative treatment of malignant extrahepatic biliary obstruction. AJR Am J Roentgenol 2010;195(6):W463–9.

87. Kullman E, Frozanpor F, Söderlund C, et al. Covered versus uncovered self-expandable nitinol stents in the palliative treatment of malignant distal biliary obstruction: results from a randomized, multicenter study. Gastrointest Endosc 2010;72(5):915–23.

88. Krokidis M, Fanelli F, Orgera G, et al. Percutaneous treatment of malignant jaundice due to extrahepatic cholangiocarcinoma: covered Viabil stent versus uncovered Wallstents. Cardiovasc Intervent Radiol 2010;33(1):97–106.

89. Telford JJ, Carr-Locke DL, Baron TH, et al. A randomized trial comparing uncovered and partially covered self-expandable metal stents in the palliation of distal malignant biliary obstruction. Gastrointest Endosc 2010;72(5):907–14.

Expandable Metal Stents for Malignant Hilar Biliary Obstruction

Christian Gerges, MD, Brigitte Schumacher, MD,
Grischa Terheggen, MD, Horst Neuhaus, MD*

KEYWORDS

- Malignant biliary obstruction • Hilar obstruction
- Biliary metal stent • Endoscopic treatment

Causes of malignant biliary obstruction at the level of the hilum can be classified into one of 3 categories (**Box 1**).[1] The most frequent cause of malignant hilar obstruction is cholangiocarcinoma (CCA), which is the second most common primary hepatobiliary cancer after hepatocellular carcinoma and accounts for 3% of all gastrointestinal cancers worldwide.[2,3] Approximately 95% of CCAs are adenocarcinomas.[4] CCA is mainly a tumor of the elderly with peak prevalence in the seventh decade of life and affects more men than women.[5] More than 90% of patients present with painless jaundice. CCA-related risk factors are primary sclerosing cholangitis (PSC), choledochal cyst, familial polyposis, hepatolithiasis, congenital hepatic fibrosis, biliary flukes (clonorchiasis, opisthorchiasis), and a history of exposure to thorotrast.[6,7] A higher prevalence of positive anti–hepatitis C virus antibody test result and hepatolithiasis has been reported to be associated with CCA.[8–11] There is evidence of a genetic link in the development of CCA.[12–14] The most common cause of CCA in younger age (third to fifth decade) is PSC, which is located at the hilum in 8% to 40% of the cases.[15] PSC is the most common risk factor in the Western countries. Differentiating between hilar CCA (HCCA) and chronic inflammatory benign hilar strictures in patients with PSC can be extremely difficult.[16]

The most common location of CCA is the main confluence of the hepatic ducts in 60% to 70% of the cases, the distal common bile duct in 20% to 30% cases, and the intrahepatic ducts in 5% to 10% cases.[7] CCA can be anatomically classified as

This work was not supported.

The authors have nothing to disclose.

Department of Internal Medicine, Evangelisches Krankenhaus Düsseldorf, Kirchfeldstraße 40, 40217 Duesseldorf, Germany

* Corresponding author. Department of Gastroenterology, Evangelisches Krankenhaus Duesseldorf, Kirchfeldstraße 40, 40217 Duesseldorf, Germany.

E-mail address: horst.neuhaus@evk-duesseldorf.de

Gastrointest Endoscopy Clin N Am 21 (2011) 481–497

doi:10.1016/j.giec.2011.04.004

1052-5157/11/$ – see front matter © 2011 Elsevier Inc. All rights reserved.

Box 1
Causes of malignant biliary strictures at the level of the hilum

1. Primary Tumors (cholangiocarcinomas)
2. Local extension (gallbladder cancer, hepatocarcinoma, pancreatic cancer)
3. Lymph node metastases (breast, colon, stomach, ovaries, lymphoma, melanoma)

---

intrahepatic (peripheral), perihilar, or extrahepatic.[17,18] This classification is important because some of the risk factors are associated with certain locations, for example, hepatolithiasis is more commonly associated with peripheral CCA than with HCCA.[19] The Japanese Liver Cancer Group described different types of tumor growth, with the infiltrating type being the most common at the perihilar region.[20] Infiltrating perihilar lesions are described as Klatskin tumors with an incidence of 1.2 per 100,000 individuals in the United States.[21] Bismuth and Corlette classified malignant hilar stenoses into 4 categories depending on the involvement of the main hepatic ducts and central segmental ducts (**Box 2; Fig. 1**).[22,23]

Differentiation between malignant and benign hilar strictures can be difficult but is important for interdisciplinary planning of treatment. The best endoscopic retrograde cholangiography (ERC)-related results can be achieved through the combination of cytologic sampling (eg, biliary brushing) and endoluminal biopsies with a sensitivity of 40% to 60%.[1,24] Newer cytologic techniques such as digital image analysis and fluorescence in situ hybridization may improve the cytologic accuracy for diagnosing CCA.[25] Endoscopic ultrasound–guided fine-needle aspiration or cholangioscopic targeted biopsies can be useful in selected cases but have not gained wide acceptance.[26–28]

Because of late clinical symptoms, patients with CCA usually present at an advanced stage of disease and/or have significant comorbidities so that not more than 10% to 20% are candidates for a potential curative surgery.[29,30] For this reason, palliative treatment plays a major role in the therapy for HCCA. The main aim is to achieve effective biliary decompression for improvement of the liver function and reduction of the risk of cholangitis. For palliation, endoscopic or percutaneous drainage are usually preferred over surgical procedures because they are less invasive.[31] Endoscopic biliary drainage of malignant hilar strictures is often more challenging and complex than management of distal malignant biliary obstruction. In particular, complete drainage of advanced hilar stenoses can be technically very demanding.[32,33] Nevertheless, endoscopic and percutaneous transhepatic stent implantations have become the standard procedures for palliation of malignant hilar obstruction. In this context, self-expandable metal stents (SEMS) offer several advantages over plastic prostheses. However, the safety and efficacy of their implantation

---

Box 2
The Bismuth-Corlette classification of malignant HCCA (see Fig. 1)

- Type I: strictures involve the proximal common hepatic duct and spare the confluence of the left and right ductal systems
- Type II: strictures involve the confluence and spare the segmental hepatic ducts
- Types IIIa and IIIb: strictures involve the right and left segmental hepatic ducts, respectively
- Type IV: strictures involve the confluence and both the right and left segmental hepatic ducts

Data from Bismuth H, Corlette MB. Intrahepatic cholangioenteric anastomosis in carcinoma of the hilus of the liver. Surg Gynecol Obstet 1975;140:170–8.

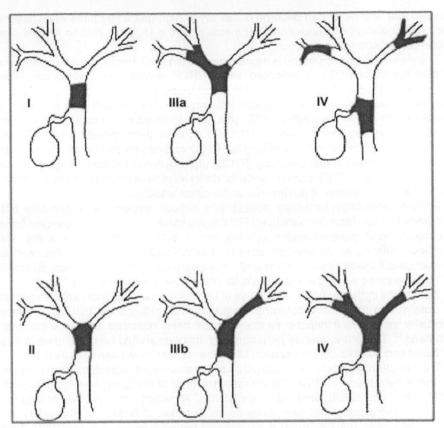

Fig. 1. Bismuth-Corlette classification (see **Box 2**).

depend on several factors, such as the anatomy of hilar stenoses, the type of stents, the technique of insertion, and the management of technical problems or complications.

ENDOSCOPIC VERSUS PERCUTANEOUS TRANSHEPATIC APPROACH

Endoscopic and percutaneous techniques allow access to hilar stenoses for subsequent diagnostic and therapeutic procedures. Both methods have advantages and disadvantages. Prophylactic administration of antibiotics is mandatory before any intervention for hilar decompression because of an increased risk of cholangitis, particularly in case of incomplete drainage.

Endoscopic retrograde cholangiopancreatography (ERCP) is recommended as the first-line drainage procedure for the palliation of jaundice in patients with inoperable tumors of Bismuth types I to III.[34] It is less invasive than the percutaneous approach but can be technically more difficult depending on local expertise with both methods. ERCP is associated with a significant risk of cholangitis after contrast injection if there is inadequate drainage of opacified ducts. Therefore, preoperative magnetic resonance cholangiopancreaticography (MRCP) is strongly recommended to plan the strategy for drainage to avoid ducts that cannot be drained.[35,36] Decompression of the dominant obstructed liver lobe usually provides adequate palliation even in patients with Bismuth type II to III stenoses. Bilateral decompression or drainage of several liver segments can become necessary in high-grade strictures when patients develop cholangitis in undrained segments or if the jaundice fails to resolve after incomplete decompression.

The percutaneous approach is more invasive than ERC. Percutaneous transhepatic cholangiography (PTC) is indicated when MRCP reveals that appropriate biliary drainage by means of ERCP can most likely not be obtained or if endoscopic drainage had failed, particularly in patients with Klatskin tumor of Bismuth type III or IV.[37] In patients with biliary obstruction, PTC should be followed by percutaneous transhepatic cholangiographic drainage (PTCD) to achieve decompression of the biliary tree and to reduce the risk of cholangitis. PTCD and can be combined with percutaneous transhepatic cholangioscopy (PTCS), photodynamic therapy (PDT), and biliary stent placement.[38] PTCS can be useful for differentiation of benign and malignant hilar strictures and insertion of guidewires under direct visual control.[39,40]

Another possibility for biliary access in a difficult anatomy is to combine both methods in a rendezvous maneuver. For this approach, a guidewire is inserted transhepatically and grasped endoscopically with a basket catheter or a snare. This method achieves an endoscopic approach to the biliary tract without the need for further percutaneous interventions and can be particularly helpful in advanced stages of hilar stenoses when there is a need for placement of several stents.[34]

Successful initial drainage, regardless of the procedure, is the most important factor in determining the clinical outcome. Retrospective studies show that ERCP-related mortality increases if hepatic segments have been opacified without subsequent drainage.[41] Therefore, rescue percutaneous drainage should be considered in case of failed endoscopic decompression of segments that have been opacified.

The selection criteria for endoscopic or percutaneous drainage depend on anatomic factors determined by MRCP, the estimated number of stents required for appropriate biliary decompression, and local experience. A recent retrospective comparison between endoscopic and percutaneous implantation of SEMS for Bismuth type III and IV stenoses demonstrated a significantly higher success rate for PTCD. There was no significant difference in terms of the incidence of cholangitis, overall complications, procedure-related mortality, and stent patency. Survival was significantly longer in those with successful drainage independent of the type of intervention.[37]

TYPES OF STENT

Biliary decompression of hilar obstruction can be obtained with plastic stents or SEMS. Straight, slightly curved, or pigtail stents are the most commonly used types of plastic endoprostheses. They are less expensive than metal stents but have a higher risk of an early occlusion with the consequence of recurrent jaundice and cholangitis. If signs of cholangitis develop, stent replacement is necessary to avoid the development of life-threatening sepsis.[42] Stent occlusion is associated with additional days of hospitalization and antibiotic therapy, and a higher number of reinterventions.[43] Attempts to increase the patency of plastic stents, such as by administration of antibiotics and/or ursodeoxycholic acid and by the use of different materials and special coatings, do not lead to significant improvement in patency.[44–47] Plastic stent patency depends not only on the material but also on the diameter, which is limited to 12F because larger devices cannot be inserted through the instrumentation channel of a standard therapeutic duodenoscope.[33] Several uncontrolled studies have shown that SEMS have a lower obstruction rate than plastic stents in patients with proximal common bile duct stenosis.[34,40,49] The median patency of metal stents was 8.9 months for patients with primary bile duct tumors and 5.4 months for all patients, and this advantage was not related to the Bismuth classification.[50] SEMS are cost-effective for patients who survive for at least 3 to 6 months.[43,51] Therefore metal stents should be considered for patients with a longer survival expectancy.[50,52] The most common causes of metal stent occlusion are growth of hyperplastic and/or tumor tissue through the lattice of the metal mesh and tumor overgrowth.

A variety of uncovered SEMS are commercially available. They mainly differ in size and material that the wire mesh is composed of. The effect of these parameters on clinical outcome is difficult to determine because of a lack of formal comparative trials. Predeployed SEMS are mounted on 6F to 8F catheters. After positioning and release, the stent diameter increases to 8 to 10 mm. Over time, the open mesh is subsequently covered by biliary epithelial cells. In contrast to plastic stents, repositioning or removal of uncovered SEMS is difficult or impossible once they have been deployed, which is why SEMS should only be used in patients with proven malignancy and unresectable tumors or in nonoperative patients. Fully covered SEMS are not indicated for proximal biliary obstruction because they may occlude the contralateral biliary system or biliary side branches. When fully expanded, nearly all commercially available SEMS have diameters of 8 or 10 mm and lengths between 4 and 10 cm. The selection depends on ductal diameter, number of SEMS required, and length of stenoses. The Wallstent (Boston Scientific, Natick, MA, USA) is a metal stent consisting of a stainless steel alloy tubular mesh. The stent length on the delivery catheter decreases by about 30% (foreshortening) after release, which has to be considered for correct positioning. The biliary Wallflex stent (Boston Scientific) is a braided platinum core nitinol stent with less shortening than the Wallstent (**Fig. 2**). The Zilver stent (Cook Medical Inc, Bloomington, IN, USA) is also made from nitinol with a laser-cut Z-like arrangement of the meshes (**Fig. 3**). It is nonforeshortening, which facilitates precise positioning. This stent has outcomes comparable with that of Wallstent for palliative drainage of distal malignant biliary stenoses with respect to technical success, occlusion rates, and overall patency.[53] Nitinol stents conform better to the biliary anatomy than stainless steel SEMS, which is particularly important in an angulated ductal system or a tortuous anatomy. In addition to this potential advantage, a subgroup analysis of

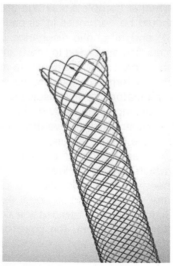

Fig. 2. SEMS for sequential implantation: braided Platinum-cored Nitinol stent (Wallflex RX biliary stent).

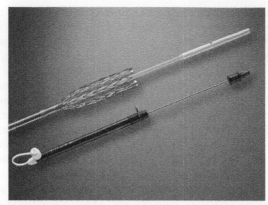

Fig. 3. SEMS for simultaneous side-by-side implantation: Nitinol stent with a 6F diameter delivery catheter (Zilver stent).

a retrospective review in 101 patients showed a significantly longer stent patency in malignant hilar stenosis with a Niti-D biliary (Taewoong Medical Co Ltd) uncovered stent as opposed to the uncovered Wallstent.[54] To date, prospective randomized controlled studies of different types of SEMS for malignant hilar obstruction have not been reported. Several strategies for prolongation of metal stent patency are currently under investigation. A pilot study indicated that the endoscopic insertion of a metal stent covered with a paclitaxel-incorporated membrane is technically feasible, safe, and effective in patients with malignant biliary obstruction.[55] Paclitaxel can suppress tissue reactions to metal stents.[56] Further studies are necessary to evaluate the adequate drug dose that exerts an antitumorous effect without damaging the adjacent normal biliary mucosa.[57]

TECHNIQUES OF IMPLANTATION AND CLINICAL RESULTS

There is controversy as to whether complete drainage of hilar obstruction is necessary. Preoperative MRCP should be performed in all patients with suspected proximal biliary stenoses. MRCP and magnetic resonance imaging (MRI) of the liver allow classification of hilar stenoses according to the Bismuth categories and determination of the volume of obstructed liver segments. In addition, it provides further information on tumor staging in terms of metastases and tumor involvement of vessels. This information is mandatory for interdisciplinary decision making in view of tumor resectability or palliation, including biliary drainage and adjunctive treatment such as PDT and/or radiochemotherapy. Palliative drainage of a Bismuth type I stricture can be achieved by a single stent because both main hepatic ducts are not involved and communicate with each other. In patients with Bismuth types II to IV, MRCP is helpful to decide which obstructed liver segments should be drained and how many stents may be needed. The endoscopic or percutaneous route should be selected depending on the anatomy and the local experience with these techniques. In most cases of Bismuth type II stenoses, a single stent placement into the right or left hepatic system is sufficient. The selection of the side depends on the volume of the obstructed liver lobe and presence or absence of atrophy. In Bismuth types III to IV obstructions, more than 1 stent can be required to achieve relief from jaundice.[58] A retrospective study in 107 patients showed that drainage of more than 50% of the liver volume seems to be an important predictor of clinical effectiveness especially in Bismuth type III strictures.[59] Recent studies suggest that the higher the degree of stenoses the more is it likely that implantation of a single stent will not achieve effective palliative drainage.[41,60] Endoscopic placement of 2 or more SEMS can be very difficult and complex. In any case, it is extremely important to avoid opacification of segments with contrast media upstream from the level of stenosis without achieving subsequent drainage because of an increased risk of cholangitis and a higher mortality rate.[41] This risk can be reduced by insertion of a guidewire toward the targeted liver lobe or an obstructed segment under fluoroscopic guidance without contrast injection. A catheter is then advanced over the wire for subsequent injection of contrast medium. After appropriate opacification showing details of the anatomy of the obstructed segment, the catheter is removed, and the guidewire remains in place. Depending on the MRCP findings and need for complete drainage, 2 or more guidewires can be placed simultaneously with the same technique. When more than 1 stent is placed, all strictures should be balloon dilated to 6 mm to facilitate placement of stents and allow a rapid expansion. The technique of implantation of more than 1 stent depends on the type of SEMS. Wallstents or Wallflex stents can be sequentially inserted and released because the smooth outer surface allows insertion of further stents alongside a released stent (**Fig. 4**). This technique should not be tried with Zilver stents because the laser-cut metallic filaments of a delivered stent may prevent advancement of another stent alongside of it. However the 6F diameter delivery catheters allow the parallel insertion of 2 predeployed stents through the working channel of a therapeutic endoscope. After correct positioning, 2 stents can then be stepwise and simultaneously released (**Fig. 5**). In patients in whom hilar stenoses do not involve the common bile duct, SEMS do not need to extend through the papilla (see **Fig. 4**). However, reinterventions may become more difficult with complete intraductal positioning. For this purpose, it is important to position the distal ends of stents next to each other so that each lumen can be individually cannulated in case of need of reintervention (see **Fig. 5**). An alternative to side-by-side stent placement is the stent-through-stent technique. It was initially described when using the Wallstent, but it can be very difficult using these stents because of the tight wire mesh.[54] In contrast, the recently developed dedicated nitinol stents have a widened mesh structure in the midsection of the stent, which facilitates insertion of a second guidewire through this section, such as into the contralateral liver lobe or another obstructed segment followed by implantation of a second stent (**Fig. 6**).[61]

Uncontrolled series indicate that implantation of SEMS can be achieved in most patients with malignant hilar obstruction.[62] In advanced tumor stages, complete drainage does not seem to be necessary. Over the course of the disease, biliary reintervention will be needed in about one-third of cases. There are few trials that provide data for comparison of plastic stents with SEMS or different type or number of SEMS for palliation of malignant hilar obstruction. A prospective multicenter observational cohort study compared the 30-day outcome of patients receiving plastic stents (n = 28) with that of those receiving SEMS (n = 34).[63] Although one-third of the patients had Bismuth II to IV stenoses, only 14% of patients in both groups were treated with bilateral stenting. These data reconfirm that a single stent seems to be appropriate for palliative drainage in most cases. Adverse outcomes including cholangitis, stent occlusion, migration, perforation, and/or the need for unplanned endoscopic or percutaneous reintervention occurred in 11 of 28 (39.3%) patients with plastic stents versus 4 of 34 (11.8%) with SEMS ($P = .017$). Plastic stents and serum bilirubin levels were found to be independent risk factors for the need for reintervention, although the Bismuth class and study center type were not.

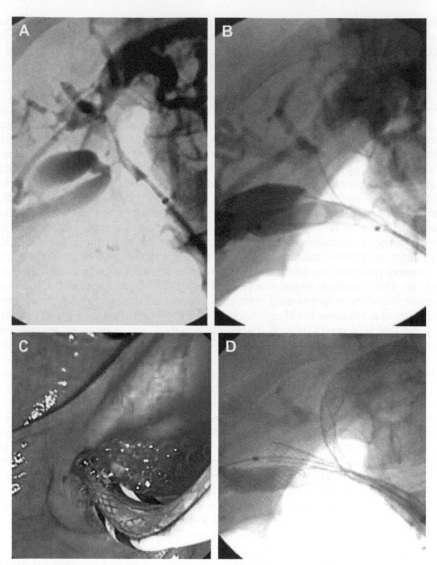

Fig. 4. (*A*) Malignant Bismuth type IIIa stenoses. (*B*) Placement of 3 hydrophilic guidewires; subsequent balloon dilatation of strictures. (*C*) Insertion of a first delivery catheter for implantation of a Wallstent into the left hepatic duct alongside the 2 other guidewires. (*D*) Complete biliary drainage after sequential parallel implantation of 3 SEMS.

COMPLICATIONS AND MANAGEMENT

ERCP may cause complications related to the biliary access and endoscopic sphincterotomy, which is usually required for diagnostic measures and stent placement, particularly for positioning more than 1 stent. However, early complications are mainly caused by cholangitis, with an incidence of 10% to 30%.[37,49,63] A significantly higher risk occurs if opacified obstructed segments cannot be subsequently drained.[41] Because of an increased mortality, a rescue percutaneous transhepatic approach should be considered in such patients. Limitations of a primary transhepatic approach

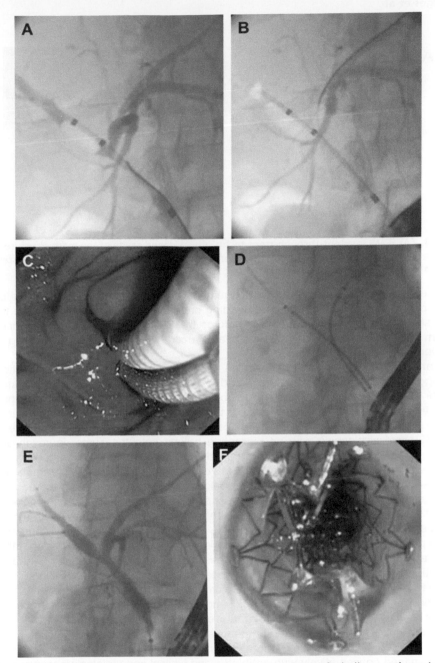

Fig. 5. (*A, B*) Malignant Bismuth type IIIa stenoses; after insertion of a balloon catheter into the right hepatic duct, the guidewire was pulled back through the site port 6 cm below the distal end of the catheter (radiopaque marker); subsequent further insertion alongside the catheter allows bouncing the hydrophilic tip of the wire against the blocked balloon of the right hepatic duct and entering into the left hepatic duct, a second wire can then be inserted through the balloon catheter into the right site. (*C, D*) Parallel and simultaneous insertion of 2 SEMS with 6F diameter delivery catheters (Zilver) into the right and left hepatic duct. (*E, F*) Complete biliary drainage after simultaneous delivery of both stents with their distal ends in midsection of the common bile duct; peroral cholangioscopy demonstrates parallel positioning of the widely opened stents ends.

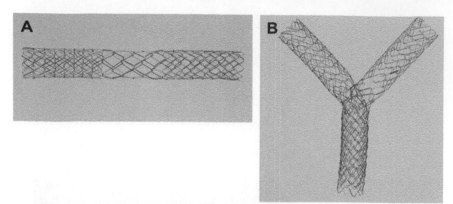

Fig. 6. (*A*) SEMS for stent-through-stent technique: widened cavity of the mesh structure in midsection of the first stent (Niti-S Y-type stent; Taewoong Medical Co Ltd). (*B*) Second stent inserted through the midsection of the first SEMS.

are related to longer hospital stay, management of a percutaneous drainage catheter, and potential complications due to bleeding or seeding of tumor cells alongside the transhepatic tract.[39] To reduce the risk of these complications, an experienced team of endoscopists and radiologists and a careful monitoring and follow-up of patients are needed.

Late stent occlusion of SEMS can be caused by hyperplastic mucosal reaction, exaggerated inflammatory reaction, and extensive fibrosis.[64–66] In approximately 20% of patients, stent occlusion can occur because of ingrowth of tumor or hyperplastic tissue through the open mesh of the stent or above or below the stent ends (overgrowth).[64,65,67,68] When occlusion occurs, SEMS can be cleared of stone material by mechanical cleaning with an extraction balloon catheter. Tumor ingrowth and hyperplastic tissue can be treated with an electrocoagulation probe or argon plasma coagulation. However, most cases of SEMS occlusion are managed by implantation of a standard polyethylene stent or an additional uncovered metal stent through the occluded SEMS.[64,69–73] Placement of a second SEMS through the existing occluded SEMS is superior to other techniques in terms of the reocclusion rate, with a 50% decrease in the need for subsequent ERCP, a trend toward longer survival compared with plastic stent and mechanical balloon cleaning,[74] and is also more cost effective. Migration of uncovered SEMS is much less common when compared with that of plastic stents because they become embedded in the bile duct wall. Several techniques such as the use of forceps and snare,[75] suture cutting device,[76] open biopsy forceps technique,[77] rat tooth forceps,[78] and coagulation and piecemeal extraction[79] have been used to manage distal migration of biliary SEMS and removal of a malfunctioning stent. Perforations related to stents are rare but may cause serious complications such as biliary peritonitis. Contained and small retroperitoneal perforations may be managed conservatively with antibiotics and clinical and radiologic observation if detected early after stent removal. There should be a low threshold for aggressive surgery when conservative management fails.[80]

ALTERNATIVE THERAPY

If preoperative staging indicates tumor resectability, a complete resection offers the only chance for cure of CCA (**Boxes 3** and **4**). It is technically demanding to achieve curative resection with histologically negative margins. This is because of the

---

Box 3
Criteria for irresectability of HCCA

1. Hepatic duct involvement up to secondary biliary radicals bilaterally.

2. Encasement or occlusion of the main portal vein proximal to its bifurcation.[a]

3. Atrophy of 1 hepatic lobe with encasement of the contralateral portal vein branch.

4. Atrophy of 1 hepatic lobe with encasement of the contralateral secondary biliary radicals.

5. Distant metastases.

[a] Relative criteria because of the possibility of performing portal vein resection and reconstruction.

Data from Jarnagin WR, Fong Y, DeMatteo RP, et al. Staging, resectability, and outcome in 225 patients with hilar cholangiocarcinoma. Ann Surg 2001;234:507–17 [discussion: 517–9].

---

anatomic location of the tumor at the biliary confluence and the vascular supply of the liver. Furthermore, the tumor has the tendency to grow into the surrounding perineural and hepatic tissue. Because only very poor survival rates after liver transplantation are achieved outside of specialized protocols in selected patients, HCCA is usually considered a contraindication for liver transplantation.[81–83] However, orthotopic liver transplantation combined with neoadjuvant chemoradiation therapy in patients with unresectable localized HCCA and without regional lymph node metastases had an 82% 5-year survival rate.[84]

In case of a palliative treatment, endoscopic or percutaneous implantation of SEMS is considered the treatment of choice. Adjunctive therapeutic approaches are external beam radiotherapy and intraluminal brachytherapy. In combination with SEMS, intraluminal brachytherapy can prolong stent patency and improve survival.[85,86] There is no standard chemotherapy protocol for HCCA, but several studies have reported a beneficial effect of the combination of chemotherapy and radiotherapy.[87] A current study compared cisplatin plus gemcitabine versus gemcitabine only for patients with locally advanced or metastatic biliary tract cancer. Patients who underwent cisplatin plus gemcitabine therapy had a higher median overall survival time (11.7 months vs 8.2 months) and median progression-free survival (8.0 months vs 5.0 months). Biliary

---

Box 4
Proposed T-stage criteria for HCCA: this preoperative staging system classifies patients according to the degree of resectability rates and survival, which is more accurate than the Bismuth-Corlette system

- T1: tumor involving biliary confluence ± unilateral extension to secondary biliary radicals.

- T2: tumor involving biliary confluence ± unilateral extension to secondary biliary radicals and ipsilateral portal vein involvement ± ipsilateral hepatic lobe atrophy.

- T3: tumor involving biliary confluence + bilateral extension to secondary biliary radicals, unilateral extension to secondary biliary radicals with contralateral portal vein involvement, unilateral extension to secondary biliary radicals with contralateral hepatic lobe atrophy, or main or bilateral portal vein involvement.

Data from Jarnagin WR, Fong Y, DeMatteo RP, et al. Staging, resectability, and outcome in 225 patients with hilar cholangiocarcinoma. Ann Surg 2001;234:507–17 [discussion: 517–9], and Hemming AW, Reed AI, Fujita S, et al. Surgical management of hilar cholangiocarcinoma. Ann Surg 2005;241:693–9 [discussion: 699–702].

stenting can also be combined with PDT to destroy cancer and neovascular cells and remodel the tumor mass.[15,88] This might prevent tumor ingrowth or overgrowth and enhance or prolong the decompressive effect of SEMS. PDT is based on the activation of photosensitizer agents (porfimer sodium [Photofrin]) after their accumulation in tumor tissue. Photofrin is a purified form of hematoporphyrin derivative that reaches its maximum concentration in tumor cells 48 hours after application. The photosensitizer can be activated with appropriate wavelength of light (630 nm for Photofrin) to generate free radicals and singlet oxygen, which are toxic to tumor cells. The combination of stenting with PDT seems to increase survival in patients with unresectable CCA campared with stenting alone.[89–91] In 2003, a prospective randomized multicenter study was terminated prematurely because PDT proved to be so superior to simple stenting treatment that further randomization was deemed unethical.[90] The results of this single-center trial are promising, but, to date, it is the only study that showed a significant survival benefit for PDT. This approach is expensive and complex and usually requires repeated interventions. In spite of promising data, it has not yet gained wide acceptance. A prospective multicenter randomized controlled trial seems to be mandatory for further evaluation.

SUMMARY

Most malignant hilar stenoses are caused by CCA. Most patients present at an advanced stage of disease with no option for a potentially curative surgical resection of the tumor. Therefore palliative treatment plays a major role in the management of HCCA. Effective biliary decompression is of great importance for improvement in liver function and treatment of associated cholangitis. Interdisciplinary planning of endoscopic and/or percutaneous transhepatic interventions should be done with consideration of the biliary anatomy determined by MRCP, risk factors of the individual patient, and local expertise with these often-complex drainage techniques. Endoscopic stent implantation is less invasive than the percutaneous approach and should be considered as the first-line drainage procedure in most of the patients with malignant hilar tumors. After successful endoscopic access to biliary obstruction, implantation of SEMS offers advantages over plastic endoprostheses in terms of stent patency and number of reinterventions. The need for a complete biliary drainage in patients with Bismuth II to IV stenoses remains controversial. A single stent seems to be appropriate in most cases, provided that undrained segments have not been opacified with contrast material. Incomplete drainage with SEMS may result in insufficient improvement of the liver function or cholangitis from undrained segments. Because uncovered SEMS are nonremovable, further stents need to be inserted through the previously placed stent when occlusion occurs, which can be technically difficult and may require transhepatic interventions. Appropriate biliary drainage with SEMS promises prolongation of survival in patients with hilar tumors, although this has not been shown in formal trials. Adjunctive treatment such as PDT, chemotherapy, and/or radiotherapy should be considered.

REFERENCES

1. Larghi A, Tringali A, Lecca PG, et al. Management of hilar biliary strictures. Am J Gastroenterol 2008;103:458–73.
2. Khan SA, Taylor-Robinson SD, Toledano MB, et al. Changing international trends in mortality rates for liver, biliary and pancreatic tumours. J Hepatol 2002;37: 806–13.

3. Vauthey JN, Blumgart LH. Recent advances in the management of cholangiocarcinomas. Semin Liver Dis 1994;14:109–14.
4. Singh P, Patel T. Advances in the diagnosis, evaluation and management of cholangiocarcinoma. Curr Opin Gastroenterol 2006;22:294–9.
5. Bloom CM, Langer B, Wilson SR. Role of US in the detection, characterization, and staging of cholangiocarcinoma. Radiographics 1999;19:1199–218.
6. Lee JH, Yang HM, Bak UB, et al. Promoting role of Clonorchis sinensis infection on induction of cholangiocarcinoma during two-step carcinogenesis. Korean J Parasitol 1994;32:13–8.
7. Okuda K, Nakanuma Y, Miyazaki M. Cholangiocarcinoma: recent progress. Part 1: epidemiology and etiology. J Gastroenterol Hepatol 2002;17:1049–55.
8. Donato F, Gelatti U, Tagger A, et al. Intrahepatic cholangiocarcinoma and hepatitis C and B virus infection, alcohol intake, and hepatolithiasis: a case-control study in Italy. Cancer Causes Control 2001;12:959–64.
9. Chen MF, Jan YY, Wang CS, et al. A reappraisal of cholangiocarcinoma in patient with hepatolithiasis. Cancer 1993;71:2461–5.
10. Chow LT, Ahuja AT, Kwong KH, et al. Mucinous cholangiocarcinoma: an unusual complication of hepatolithiasis and recurrent pyogenic cholangitis. Histopathology 1997;30:491–4.
11. Chang KY, Chang JY, Yen Y. Increasing incidence of intrahepatic cholangiocarcinoma and its relationship to chronic viral hepatitis. J Natl Compr Canc Netw 2009; 7:423–7.
12. Levi S, Urbano-Ispizua A, Gill R, et al. Multiple K-ras codon 12 mutations in cholangiocarcinomas demonstrated with a sensitive polymerase chain reaction technique. Cancer Res 1991;51:3497–502.
13. Okuda K, Nakanuma Y, Miyazaki M. Cholangiocarcinoma: recent progress. Part 2: molecular pathology and treatment. J Gastroenterol Hepatol 2002;17: 1056–63.
14. Khan SA, Thomas HC, Toledano MB, et al. p53 Mutations in human cholangiocarcinoma: a review. Liver Int 2005;25:704–16.
15. Khan SA, Thomas HC, Davidson BR, et al. Cholangiocarcinoma. Lancet 2005; 366:1303–14.
16. van Leeuwen DJ, Reeders JW. Primary sclerosing cholangitis and cholangiocarcinoma as a diagnostic and therapeutic dilemma. Ann Oncol 1999;10(Suppl 4): 89–93.
17. Nakeeb A, Pitt HA, Sohn TA, et al. Cholangiocarcinoma. A spectrum of intrahepatic, perihilar, and distal tumors. Ann Surg 1996;224:463–73 [discussion: 473–5].
18. Meyer DG, Weinstein BJ. Klatskin tumors of the bile ducts: sonographic appearance. Radiology 1983;148:803–4.
19. Su CH, Shyr YM, Lui WY, et al. Hepatolithiasis associated with cholangiocarcinoma. Br J Surg 1997;84:969–73.
20. The general rules for the clinical and pathological study of primary liver cancer. Liver Cancer Study Group of Japan. Jpn J Surg 1989;19:98–129.
21. Klatskin G. Adenocarcinoma of the hepatic duct at its bifurcation within the porta hepatis. An unusual tumor with distinctive clinical and pathological features. Am J Med 1965;38:241–56.
22. Bismuth H, Corlette MB. Intrahepatic cholangioenteric anastomosis in carcinoma of the hilus of the liver. Surg Gynecol Obstet 1975;140:170–8.
23. Bismuth H, Castaing D, Traynor O. Resection or palliation: priority of surgery in the treatment of hilar cancer. World J Surg 1988;12:39–47.

24. De Bellis M, Sherman S, Fogel EL, et al. Tissue sampling at ERCP in suspected malignant biliary strictures (Part 1). Gastrointest Endosc 2002;56: 552–61.
25. Chahal P, Baron TH. Endoscopic palliation of cholangiocarcinoma. Curr Opin Gastroenterol 2006;22:551–60.
26. Tsuyuguchi T, Fukuda Y, Saisho H. Peroral cholangioscopy for the diagnosis and treatment of biliary diseases. J Hepatobiliary Pancreat Surg 2006;13:94–9.
27. DeWitt J, Misra VL, Leblanc JK, et al. EUS-guided FNA of proximal biliary strictures after negative ERCP brush cytology results. Gastrointest Endosc 2006;64: 325–33.
28. Baron TH. Palliation of malignant obstructive jaundice. Gastroenterol Clin North Am 2006;35:101–12.
29. Jarnagin WR, Fong Y, DeMatteo RP, et al. Staging, resectability, and outcome in 225 patients with hilar cholangiocarcinoma. Ann Surg 2001;234:507–17 [discussion: 517–9].
30. Prat F, Chapat O, Ducot B, et al. A randomized trial of endoscopic drainage methods for inoperable malignant strictures of the common bile duct. Gastrointest Endosc 1998;47:1–7.
31. Singhal D, van Gulik TM, Gouma DJ. Palliative management of hilar cholangiocarcinoma. Surg Oncol 2005;14:59–74.
32. Ducreux M, Liguory C, Lefebvre JF, et al. Management of malignant hilar biliary obstruction by endoscopy. Results and prognostic factors. Dig Dis Sci 1992; 37:778–83.
33. Liu CL, Lo CM, Lai EC, et al. Endoscopic retrograde cholangiopancreatography and endoscopic endoprosthesis insertion in patients with Klatskin tumors. Arch Surg 1998;133:293–6.
34. Lee SH, Park JK, Yoon WJ, et al. Optimal biliary drainage for inoperable Klatskin's tumor based on Bismuth type. World J Gastroenterol 2007;13:3948–55.
35. Hintze RE, Abou-Rebyeh H, Adler A, et al. Magnetic resonance cholangio pancreatography-guided unilateral endoscopic stent placement for Klatskin tumors. Gastrointest Endosc 2001;53:40–6.
36. Freeman ML, Overby C. Selective MRCP and CT-targeted drainage of malignant hilar biliary obstruction with self-expanding metallic stents. Gastrointest Endosc 2003;58:41–9.
37. Paik WH, Park YS, Hwang JH, et al. Palliative treatment with self-expandable metallic stents in patients with advanced type III or IV hilar cholangiocarcinoma: a percutaneous versus endoscopic approach. Gastrointest Endosc 2009;69: 55–62.
38. Charton JP, Shim C, Neuhaus H. Percutaneous transhepatic cholangiography and cholangioskopy. In: Classen M, Tytgat GNJ, Lightdale CJ, editors. Gastroenterological endoscopy. 2nd edition. New York: Thieme; 2010. p. 167–76.
39. Itoi T, Neuhaus H, Chen YK. Diagnostic value of image-enhanced video cholangiopancreatoscopy. Gastrointest Endosc Clin N Am 2009;19:557–66.
40. Seo DW, Kim MH, Lee SK, et al. Usefulness of cholangioscopy in patients with focal stricture of the intrahepatic duct unrelated to intrahepatic stones. Gastrointest Endosc 1999;49:204–9.
41. Chang WH, Kortan P, Haber GB. Outcome in patients with bifurcation tumors who undergo unilateral versus bilateral hepatic duct drainage. Gastrointest Endosc 1998;47:354–62.
42. Motte S, Deviere J, Dumonceau JM, et al. Risk factors for septicemia following endoscopic biliary stenting. Gastroenterology 1991;101:1374–81.

43. Kaassis M, Boyer J, Dumas R, et al. Plastic or metal stents for malignant stricture of the common bile duct? Results of a randomized prospective study. Gastrointest Endosc 2003;57:178–82.

44. Libby ED, Leung JW. Prevention of biliary stent clogging: a clinical review. Am J Gastroenterol 1996;91:1301–8.

45. Terruzzi V, Comin U, De Grazia F, et al. Prospective randomized trial comparing Tannenbaum Teflon and standard polyethylene stents in distal malignant biliary stenosis. Gastrointest Endosc 2000;51:23–7.

46. Costamagna G, Mutignani M, Rotondano G, et al. Hydrophilic hydromer-coated polyurethane stents versus uncoated stents in malignant biliary obstruction: a randomized trial. Gastrointest Endosc 2000;51:8–11.

47. Catalano MF, Geenen JE, Lehman GA, et al. "Tannenbaum" Teflon stents versus traditional polyethylene stents for treatment of malignant biliary stricture. Gastrointest Endosc 2002;55:354–8.

48. Peters RA, Williams SG, Lombard M, et al. The management of high-grade hilar strictures by endoscopic insertion of self-expanding metal endoprostheses. Endoscopy 1997;29:10–6.

49. Cheng JL, Bruno MJ, Bergman JJ, et al. Endoscopic palliation of patients with biliary obstruction caused by nonresectable hilar cholangiocarcinoma: efficacy of self-expandable metallic Wallstents. Gastrointest Endosc 2002;56:33–9.

50. Cipolletta L, Rotondano G, Marmo R, et al. Endoscopic palliation of malignant obstructive jaundice: an evidence-based review. Dig Liver Dis 2007;39:375–88.

51. Schmassmann A, von Gunten E, Knuchel J, et al. Wallstents versus plastic stents in malignant biliary obstruction: effects of stent patency of the first and second stent on patient compliance and survival. Am J Gastroenterol 1996;91:654–9.

52. Soderlund C, Linder S. Covered metal versus plastic stents for malignant common bile duct stenosis: a prospective, randomized, controlled trial. Gastrointest Endosc 2006;63:986–95.

53. Loew BJ, Howell DA, Sanders MK, et al. Comparative performance of uncoated, self-expanding metal biliary stents of different designs in 2 diameters: final results of an international multicenter, randomized, controlled trial. Gastrointest Endosc 2009;70:445–53.

54. Neuhaus H, Gottlieb K, Classen M. The "stent through wire mesh technique" for complicated biliary strictures. Gastrointest Endosc 1993;39:553–6.

55. Suk KT, Kim JW, Kim HS, et al. Human application of a metallic stent covered with a paclitaxel-incorporated membrane for malignant biliary obstruction: multicenter pilot study. Gastrointest Endosc 2007;66:798–803.

56. Rowinsky EK, Donehower RC. Paclitaxel (taxol). N Engl J Med 1995;332:1004–14.

57. Lee SS, Shin JH, Han JM, et al. Histologic influence of paclitaxel-eluting covered metallic stents in a canine biliary model. Gastrointest Endosc 2009;69:1140–7.

58. Inal M, Akgul E, Aksungur E, et al. Percutaneous placement of biliary metallic stents in patients with malignant hilar obstruction: unilobar versus bilobar drainage. J Vasc Interv Radiol 2003;14:1409–16.

59. Vienne A, Hobeika E. Prediction of drainage effectiveness during endoscopic stenting of malignant hilar strictures: the role of liver volume assessment. Gastrointest Endosc 2010;72:728–35.

60. Naitoh I, Ohara H, Nakazawa T, et al. Unilateral versus bilateral endoscopic metal stenting for malignant hilar biliary obstruction. J Gastroenterol Hepatol 2009;24:552–7.

61. Park do H, Lee SS, Moon JH, et al. Newly designed stent for endoscopic bilateral stent-in-stent placement of metallic stents in patients with malignant hilar biliary strictures: multicenter prospective feasibility study (with videos). Gastrointest Endosc 2009;69:1357–60.

62. Rey JF, Dumas R, Canard JM, et al. Guidelines of the French Society of Digestive Endoscopy: biliary stenting. Endoscopy 2002;34:169–73, 181–5.

63. Perdue DG, Freeman ML, DiSario JA, et al. Plastic versus self-expanding metallic stents for malignant hilar biliary obstruction: a prospective multicenter observational cohort study. J Clin Gastroenterol 2008;42:1040–6.

64. Knyrim K, Wagner HJ, Pausch J, et al. A prospective, randomized, controlled trial of metal stents for malignant obstruction of the common bile duct. Endoscopy 1993;25:207–12.

65. Bethge N, Wagner HJ, Knyrim K, et al. Technical failure of biliary metal stent deployment in a series of 116 applications. Endoscopy 1992;24:395–400.

66. Huibregtse K, Carr-Locke DL, Cremer M, et al. Biliary stent occlusion–a problem solved with self-expanding metal stents? European Wallstent Study Group. Endoscopy 1992;24:391–4.

67. Raijman I. Biliary and pancreatic stents. Gastrointest Endosc Clin N Am 2003;13: 561–92, vii–viii.

68. Davids PH, Groen AK, Rauws EA, et al. Randomised trial of self-expanding metal stents versus polyethylene stents for distal malignant biliary obstruction. Lancet 1992;340:1488–92.

69. Donelli G, Guaglianone E, Di Rosa R, et al. Plastic biliary stent occlusion: factors involved and possible preventive approaches. Clin Med Res 2007;5:53–60.

70. Ell C, Fleig WE, Hochberger J. Broken biliary metal stent after repeated electrocoagulation for tumor ingrowth. Gastrointest Endosc 1992;38:197–9.

71. Cremer M, Deviere J, Sugai B, et al. Expandable biliary metal stents for malignancies: endoscopic insertion and diathermic cleaning for tumor ingrowth. Gastrointest Endosc 1990;36:451–7.

72. Tham TC, Carr-Locke DL, Vandervoort J, et al. Management of occluded biliary Wallstents. Gut 1998;42:703–7.

73. Lossef SV, Druy E, Jelinger E, et al. Use of hot-tip laser probes to recanalize occluded expandable metallic biliary endoprostheses. AJR Am J Roentgenol 1992;158:199–201.

74. Rogart JN, Boghos A, Rossi F, et al. Analysis of endoscopic management of occluded metal biliary stents at a single tertiary care center. Gastrointest Endosc 2008;68:676–82.

75. Familiari P, Bulajic M, Mutignani M, et al. Endoscopic removal of malfunctioning biliary self-expandable metallic stents. Gastrointest Endosc 2005;62:903–10.

76. Levy MJ, Wiersema MJ. Endoscopic removal of a biliary Wallstent with a suture-cutting device in a patient with primary pancreatic lymphoma. Endoscopy 2002; 34:835–7.

77. Matsushita M, Takakuwa H, Nishio A, et al. Open-biopsy-forceps technique for endoscopic removal of distally migrated and impacted biliary metallic stents. Gastrointest Endosc 2003;58:924–7.

78. Shin HP, Kim MH, Jung SW, et al. Endoscopic removal of biliary self-expandable metallic stents: a prospective study. Endoscopy 2006;38:1250–5.

79. Kahaleh M, Tokar J, Le T, et al. Removal of self-expandable metallic Wallstents. Gastrointest Endosc 2004;60:640–4.

80. Kundu R, Pleskow D. Biliary and pancreatic stents: complications and management. Tech Gastrointest Endosc 2007;9:125–34.

81. Iwatsuki S, Todo S, Marsh JW, et al. Treatment of hilar cholangiocarcinoma (Klatskin tumors) with hepatic resection or transplantation. J Am Coll Surg 1998;187:358–64.

82. Meyer CG, Penn I, James L. Liver transplantation for cholangiocarcinoma: results in 207 patients. Transplantation 2000;69(8):1633–7.

83. Robles R, Figueras J, Turrion VS, et al. Spanish experience in liver transplantation for hilar and peripheral cholangiocarcinoma. Ann Surg 2004;239:265–71.

84. Rea DJ, Heimbach JK, Rosen CB, et al. Liver transplantation with neoadjuvant chemoradiation is more effective than resection for hilar cholangiocarcinoma. Ann Surg 2005;242:451–8 [discussion: 458–61].

85. Bruha R, Petrtyl J, Kubecova M, et al. Intraluminal brachytherapy and selfexpandable stents in nonresectable biliary malignancies–the question of long-term palliation. Hepatogastroenterology 2001;48:631–7.

86. Kubota Y, Takaoka M, Kin H, et al. Endoscopic irradiation and parallel arrangement of Wallstents for hilar cholangiocarcinoma. Hepatogastroenterology 1998; 45:415–9.

87. Morganti AG, Trodella L, Valentini V, et al. Combined modality treatment in unresectable extrahepatic biliary carcinoma. Int J Radiat Oncol Biol Phys 2000;46: 913–9.

88. Berr F, Tannapfel A, Lamesch P, et al. Neoadjuvant photodynamic therapy before curative resection of proximal bile duct carcinoma. J Hepatol 2000;32:352–7.

89. Kahaleh M, Mishra R, Shami VM, et al. Unresectable cholangiocarcinoma: comparison of survival in biliary stenting alone versus stenting with photodynamic therapy. Clin Gastroenterol Hepatol 2008;6:290–7.

90. Ortner ME, Caca K, Berr F, et al. Successful photodynamic therapy for nonresectable cholangiocarcinoma: a randomized prospective study. Gastroenterology 2003;125:1355–63.

91. Zoepf T, Jakobs R, Arnold JC, et al. Palliation of nonresectable bile duct cancer: improved survival after photodynamic therapy. Am J Gastroenterol 2005;100: 2426–30.

Pancreatic Stents

Jacques Deviere, MD, PhD

KEYWORDS

• Pancreatic duct • Stent • Pancreatitis • Drainage

Although there are various types of stents that provide drainage and bypass for the treatment of bile duct obstruction, leaks, and stones,[1] their use in the pancreas has for long been confined and limited to referral centers that specialize in the treatment of patients with severe chronic pancreatitis (CP) and acute relapsing pancreatitis.

Therapeutic developments in endoscopic treatment of pancreatic diseases and a better understanding of the cause and prevention of endoscopic retrograde cholangiopancreatography (ERCP)–related complications have recently expanded the use of stents placed into the pancreatic duct and directly into pancreatic fluid collections (PFCs).

There are now a variety of indications for pancreatic stent placement, although some are still debated, whereas others are becoming scientifically established. Nearly all pancreatic stents are composed of plastic and inserted into the pancreatic duct. Their size, shape, and purpose vary by indication, and follow-up after placement must be tailored to the indication.

Also unique to pancreatic stents is that they are almost exclusively used for the treatment and/or prevention of benign conditions despite data to support their role in palliation of pain in selected patients with pancreatic cancer.[2,3]

This article reviews the major indications for pancreatic stent placement and focuses on the choice of stents, technique of implantation, and follow-up.

PREVENTION OF POST-ERCP PANCREATITIS

Pancreatitis remains the most common complication of ERCP and occurs after 1% to 25% of procedures. Large prospective studies have shown that its incidence varies with the type and indication of the procedure performed, patient susceptibility, and case volume of the operator.[4–7] The severity of post-ERCP pancreatitis (PEP) is much more difficult to predict. Severe PEP accounts for around 10% of all cases, and although risk factors for PEP have been identified, predictors of severe PEP are lacking. With the exception of nonsteroidal antiinflammatory drugs (100 mg of diclofenac or indomethacin administered rectally), no other drug prophylaxis of PEP pancreatitis has been proven to be effective.[8,9]

Department of Gastroenterology, Hepatopancreatology and Digestive Oncology, Erasme University Hospital, Université Libre de Bruxelles, Route de Lennik 808, B–1070 Brussels, Belgium
E-mail address: jacques.deviere@erasme.ulb.ac.be

Gastrointest Endoscopy Clin N Am 21 (2011) 499–510
doi:10.1016/j.giec.2011.04.011
1052-5157/11/$ – see front matter © 2011 Elsevier Inc. All rights reserved.

Over the last 20 years, there have been major advances in the ERCP technique to prevent PEP. These include guidewire-directed deep biliary cannulation and, more importantly, placement of prophylactic pancreatic duct stents in patients at a high risk for developing PEP.

A total of 8 randomized controlled trials (RCTs), multiple prospective uncontrolled studies, and 4 meta-analysis have compared the rates of pancreatitis after ERCP with and without prophylactic pancreatic stent placement.[10–16] Prophylactic stent placement not only reduces the incidence of PEP, particularly in high-risk patients, but also virtually eliminates severe pancreatitis.

Many studies criticize the absence of intent-to-treat analysis (patients with attempted but unsuccessful stent placement were excluded). However, a meta-analysis[13] of the 4 RCTs used intent-to-treat principles by assuming that PEP developed in patients in whom attempted prophylactic pancreatic stent placement failed, even when the clinical outcome was not stated in the original study. Despite using this approach, the odds ratio in the stent group was 0.44 compared with controls and was significantly different in favor of stent placement. On the basis of these results, prophylactic stent placement can be considered as the single most-important advance in the last 15 years for prevention of PEP in high-risk patients.

Despite these findings, questions remain as to when to place a prophylactic pancreatic stent, what type of stent to place, and what is the optimal follow-up period to ensure adequate removal.

The incidence of adverse events associated with pancreatic stent placement is around 4%[13,17] and must be considered in the decision-making process for placement of stent. Immediate complications include the potential for the guidewire to damage secondary pancreatic duct branches, possible misplacement completely into the duct, ductal perforation by the stent, or trauma caused by multiple manipulations during attempted placement. Midterm complications include stent-induced ductal alterations causing CP-like changes,[18,19] which although usually regress spontaneously, can lead to permanent damage, especially when placed in normal ducts for a prolonged period. For these reasons, traditional 5F and 7F flanged stents made of rigid polyethylene are not recommended because they (1) may induce ductal changes and (2) do not spontaneously pass out of the duct because of the presence of a proximal flap. The most frequently used stents are short, 4F to 5F in diameter, and devoid of proximal flaps (Cook Endoscopy, Winston Salem, NC, USA; Hobbs Medical Inc, Stafford Spring, CT, USA), and because they are made of newer materials they are potentially safer than the traditional polyethylene stents. Several investigators have proposed the use of long, unflanged 3F pancreatic stents that require the use of a 0.018-in guidewire. Although there is less early migration out of the duct (potentially decreasing the rate of PEP) and the procedure may be less traumatic to the duct, the additional guidewire exchange from a 0.035-in wire used for other aspects of the procedure are time consuming and can cause ductal injury. In addition, the need for negotiating tight loops in the pancreatic neck renders their placement more difficult. Two recent RCTs that compared short 5F stents with long 3F stents for the prevention of PEP did not show significant differences in PEP with the use of the 2 stents but showed that there was less spontaneous migration at 2 weeks and there were more failures of implantation when using the 3F stents.[20,21] At present, 3- to 5-cm long 5F stents without internal flanges, with an external (duodenal) pigtail or flap, are considered to be the best choice. Stent passage out of the duct (preferred to prevent the need for an additional endoscopic procedure) occurs by 2 weeks in more than 95% of the cases. A plain abdominal radiograph is necessary at that time, and the stent should be removed endoscopically if it remains (**Fig. 1**).

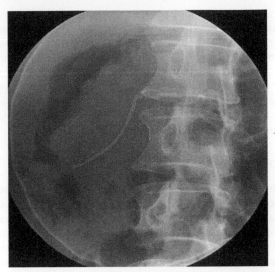

Fig. 1. A 5F, 5-cm pancreatic duct stent without internal flaps implanted for preventing PEP.

The inherent complications related to stent placement justify their use only in patients at a high risk for PEP, and they have been proved to reduce PEP in RCTs.[11,12] Stent placement is strongly recommended when technical maneuvers associated with a high risk of pancreatitis are performed as well as in those patients with a known high susceptibility for PEP (**Box 1**).

As prophylactic stenting has become part of routine practice, knowledge has also been gained to use techniques to increase the rate of successful biliary cannulation. For example, when the guidewire has passed into the pancreatic duct during repeated biliary cannulation attempts, it can be left in the duct to allow for pancreatic stent placement at the end of the procedure. The bile duct is selectively cannulated using a second guidewire preloaded into a catheter or sphincterotome.[22] Similarly, a stent can be placed into the pancreatic duct before continuing cannulation using standard techniques and to allow delineation of the sphincter anatomy for precut sphincterotomy while also reducing the risk of PEP.

Box 1
Indications for prophylactic pancreatic stent placement during ERCP

Definitive:

- Pancreatic sphincterotomy for sphincter of Oddi dysfunction/acute recurrent pancreatitis
- Ampullectomy

Highly recommended:

- Difficult biliary cannulation, involving instrumentation or injection of the pancreas
- Pancreatic sphincterotomy (major or minor)
- Aggressive instrumentation of the pancreatic duct (brush cytology, biopsies)
- Balloon dilatation of an intact biliary sphincter (balloon sphincteroplasty)
- Prior PEP
- Precut sphincterotomy starting at the papillary orifice

Despite the considerable amount of evidence supporting the use of prophylactic stents, 2 recent surveys[23,24] have shown that many endoscopists in Europe and the United States still do not attempt to place pancreatic stents in high-risk cases, citing lack of expertise as an explanation. Monitoring of PEP incidence in their center and the hospital ERCP volume of more than 500 cases per year are 2 independent factors associated with the use of prophylactic stents.[24] These results are of major interest because this observation could further increase the differences in terms of complications between low- and high-volume centers/practitioners[5] if there is a lack of proper training and awareness of prophylactic pancreatic stents.

STENTS FOR PANCREATIC STRICTURE MANAGEMENT

Dominant, symptomatic, main pancreatic duct strictures in the setting of CP are amenable to endoscopic drainage by stent insertion. Stent placement is usually performed after pancreatic sphincterotomy and fragmentation of pancreatic stones, most often using extracorporeal shock wave lithotripsy (ESWL). Underlying strictures are often present in patients with intraductal stones.[25] The technique used, the purpose of use, and the type of stents placed for resolving strictures are different from those for prevention of PEP. Because most CP strictures are tight and fibrotic, mechanical or pneumatic dilatation is often required to facilitate stent insertion. The initial dilatation is usually performed with a 4- to 6-mm dilating balloon (**Fig. 2**)

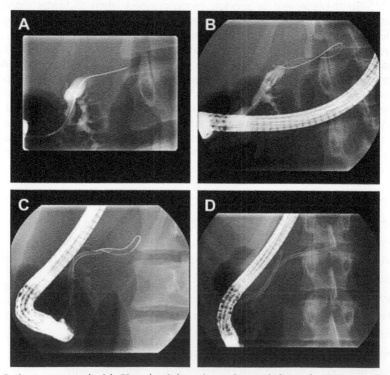

Fig. 2. Patient presented with CP and a tight stricture located above the minor papilla. After insertion of a guidewire (A), balloon dilatation is performed with a 6-mm, 4-cm hydrostatic balloon (B) and an 8.5F, 7-cm stent is placed over a FUSION (Cook Medical) introducer (C), followed by the placement of a second 8.5F, 5-cm stent (D) over the same guidewire.

depending on the size of the dilated duct upstream to the stricture and the number of stents placed.[26,27] If the stricture is too tight to allow passage of a dilating balloon catheter, an 8.5F stent retriever (Soehendra stent retriever, Cook Endoscopy) may be passed over a guidewire to allow subsequent passage of a balloon catheter.

The principle of dilation and stent placement is that decompression of the main pancreatic duct can lead to resolution of obstructive pancreatic pain. The goal of longer-term stent placement is to resolve or permanently improve the stricture diameter to an adequate size to ultimately allow stent removal without recurrence of symptoms.[26,28–31] Stents used for this indication are larger in diameter (8.5F or 10F) to remain patent as long as possible and have internal flanges to prevent outward migration.

Although surgical drainage has been shown to be more effective than endoscopic drainage in relieving pain at short-term and midterm outcomes in 2 RCTs,[27,28] multiple retrospective and prospective series have shown that endotherapy can offer pain relief in approximately 80% of patients and avoid the need for surgery in two-thirds.[25–29,32–36]

Stent placement is only a part of the treatment of CP because ESWL is often necessary when associated stones are present. Single 10F polyethylene stents are most often used, the length of which is determined by the length and location of the stenosis, with care to avoid impaction of the proximal end (tail) into the pancreatic duct. Stents are available with shapes specifically designed to conform to the anatomy of the pancreas and with multiple side holes to provide adequate drainage of secondary ducts,[37,38] although such stents have not been shown to provide a significant benefit. Wing stents with only a small internal lumen for the guidewire[39] have also been used for prolonged periods in pancreatic ducts for stricture management but without sufficient data to recommend them over traditional stent designs.

When large-bore stents are used for CP strictures, they remain in place for up to or greater than 1 year to provide adequate remodeling of the stricture and to avoid recurrence after retrieval.[28,29] In a series of 100 patients in whom stents were exchanged and remained in place for 2 years, only 30% experienced recurrent pain within 2 years of additional follow-up after stent removal.[29] Most of the patients experience pain relapse within 12 months after stent removal allowing identification of those who would have a long-term benefit from surgery.

The reported mean patency of large pancreatic stents is 6 to 12 months; therefore the need for multiple stent exchange, scheduled or on demand, represents a limitation of this treatment. Costamagna and colleagues[26] in Italy recommend an approach similar to treatment of benign biliary strictures; in this approach, as many stents as possible are placed side by side to accelerate stricture improvement/resolution. Using this approach, they were able to achieve symptomatic relief in 85% of the cases after only 7 months of stent placement at a mean follow-up of 3 years after stent removal.[26]

This multiple large-bore pancreatic stent approach is currently used in several centers dedicated to pancreatic endotherapy and might decrease the need for repeated stent exchange. It is thought that pancreatic juice is able to flow into the duodenum between the stents even when the stents are occluded. Technically, these multiple stents can be placed using a system that allows intraductal exchange (Fusion system, Cook Endoscopy), allowing the placement of multiple stents over a single guidewire after stricture dilation (see **Fig. 2**).

Large-bore pancreatic stents may also be used for the treatment of pancreatic duct leaks, particularly when the leak can be bridged. In this case, stents remain for 3 to 6 months after closure of the leak.[40,41]

Although it may be tempting to use self-expandable metal stents (SEMS), possibly fully covered, to dilate pancreatic stenoses, they have caused complications including pain, pancreatitis, stent-induced changes of the main pancreatic duct, and relapsing stenoses inside the stent when disruption of the coating occurs. Thus, SEMS for pancreatic duct use must be considered as experimental and must not be used routinely.[42,43]

STENTS PLACED FOR REROUTING PANCREATIC JUICE

With the development of therapeutic endoscopic ultrasound (EUS), almost every PFC occurring in the setting of acute pancreatitis or CP has become amenable to endoscopic therapy, including transmural drainage of nonbulging collections located close to the gastrointestinal lumen tract or near the tail of the pancreas.[44–46] Endotherapy in this indication is now not only challenging surgery but also becoming the procedure of choice, offering similar results with better cost-efficiency and quality of life.[47]

When such PFC drainage is performed, communication with the stomach or the duodenum is maintained by the placement of 1 or 2 stents. The most frequently used stents are double-pigtail 7F or 8.5F stents, which prevent dislodgement. When placed by EUS, 10F stents are much less often used because therapeutic echoendoscopes have therapeutic channel diameters of 3.7 mm instead of the 4.2 mm diameter of duodenoscopes, rendering the friction too great to allow passage, especially when multiple guidewires are placed. Therefore, the stent that is usually inserted with a therapeutic echoendoscope has a diameter of 8.5F or 9F (**Fig. 3**).

When a stent is inserted after transmural drainage, the patency of the stent is much less important than for transpapillary placement because their role is to maintain the fistula between the collection and the gastrointestinal tract, serving as a guide. When the collection communicates with the pancreatic duct because of a partial or complete rupture of the pancreatic ducts, the stents also serves as a long-term communication to maintain the alternative route for pancreatic secretions from the pancreas located above the rupture to the stomach or duodenum.[41,48]

It has long been considered that stents should be removed within 3 to 6 months after transmural PFC drainage.[45,46,49,50] The rate of PFC recurrence in these original series varied between 10% and 30% and usually occurred within a year after treatment. In an RCT[48] comparing stent removal after PFC with stents left in place for the duration of the study, the author's group showed that the rate of recurrence was significantly lower in and that most of the recurrences occurred in patients who had a disconnected tail syndrome (**Fig. 4**). Based on these data, it can be suggested that when a collection has disappeared after endotherapy, the integrity of the main pancreatic duct should be assessed (ideally by a dynamic magnetic resonance cholangio pancreatography) and, if a rupture/disconnection is seen, stents should be left in place for years.[51] Routine stent exchange is not necessary because these stents serve as a guide for flow.

As an extension to PFC drainage, stents can also be used to reroute the pancreatic juice when an external fistula is present. Indeed, this can be considered as a virtual collection, and a transmural stent will favor internal drainage instead of external fistulae (**Fig. 5**). A combined endoscopic (with EUS) and percutaneous approach may be needed in these cases.[52] EUS has not only extended the plumbing capabilities of the endoscopist toward small or large PFC but also allows, in selected cases, to create direct transmural access to the pancreatic duct by pancreaticogastrostomy or duodenostomy.[53,54] This technique is usually performed in the setting of severe obstructive pancreatitis or after pancreatic-enteric anastomosis after failure of other routes of access. Again in this case, when the anastomosis is created, the role of

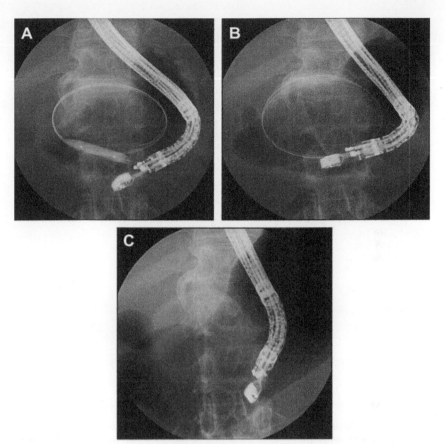

Fig. 3. Cystogastrostomy and stenting. After access to the cavity, 2 guidewires are inserted and balloon dilatation is performed (*A*). The first double-pigtail 8.5F stent is inserted over a guidewire, alongside a second one, left in place after the stent's release (*B*), and is used for the placement of a second stent (*C*).

the stent is to act as a guide to maintain the fistula tract, and usually, 7F to 9F flanged stents are chosen. At present, there are not enough data available to know whether these types of cases require maintenance of stents for years or if, similar to dominant strictures seen in CP, the stent can be removed after a certain period and the fistula tract would remain open.

TREATMENT OF INTERNAL PANCREATIC DUCT FISTULA

Patients with CP can present with large plural effusions because of pancreaticopleural fistula or with pancreatic ascites because of intra-abdominal leak. Similar to a bile leak, placement of a pancreatic stent diverts pancreatic juice from the leak site to the duodenum allowing the leak to close.[55] It is important that any obstruction (strictures) between the duodenum and papilla be bridged.

OTHER USES OF PANCREATIC DUCT STENTS

There are increasing data to show that pancreatic duct stenting allows healing of pancreatic duct injuries and leaks after trauma caused by injury[56,57] or surgery,

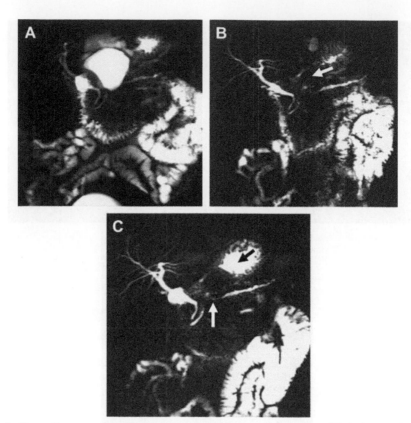

Fig. 4. Magnetic resonance imaging performed before (*A*) and after (*B*) drainage of a PFC under EUS guidance with placement of a double-pigtail stent (*arrow, B*). The dynamic magnetic resonance cholangio pancreatography with secretin injection (*C*) performed after the procedure shows the rupture of the main pancreatic duct (*white arrow, C*) and filling of the stomach by secretion from the proximal pancreas (*black arrow, C*), illustrating the new pathway for secretions provided by the stent.

deliberately (pancreatic tail resection) or inadvertently. In many of these patients, particularly children, the main pancreatic duct is otherwise normal and relatively small in caliber. Thus, smaller-diameter stents are used, at least initially, and can be upsized later, if needed.

Several studies have shown that the rate of postoperative pancreatic duct leaks after distal pancreatectomy can be prevented by preoperative endoscopic placement of pancreatic duct stents.[58,59]

STENT PLACEMENT TECHNIQUES

Pancreatic duct stents are inserted using a guidewire and pusher tube. Larger stents may have an inner guiding catheter. For 5F stents, nearly any standard accessory used during the course of an ERCP (sphincterotome, catheter, stone retrieval balloon) can be used as a pusher tube. A pancreatic sphincterotomy is not required for placing a single stent, even when a large-bore 10F stent is placed. However, for multiple stent placement, a sphincterotomy is often performed. During placement of pigtail stents, the tip of the endoscope needs to be away from the source (papilla or transmural

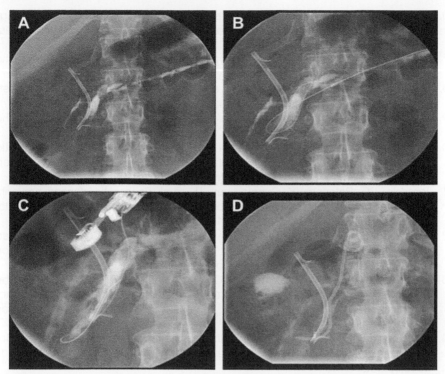

Fig. 5. Percutaneous opacification of an external fistula after severe acute pancreatitis and main pancreatic duct disruption (*A*). The virtual fistula tract is filled with contrast and saline through a percutaneous approach (*B*). The transient collection is visualized and punctured by EUS (*C*) and a transduodenal stent is implanted to re-reroute pancreatic secretions (*D*).

drainage site) during the final stage of delivery to allow the pigtail to exit the endoscope.[60]

In conclusion, stenting into or around the pancreas involves a wide spectrum of indications, mostly benign, for which the common word is that they belong to specialized multidisciplinary care. Specific pancreatic therapies should be performed in referral centers, but prophylactic pancreatic stenting has become a part of ERCP routine practice.

REFERENCES

1. Somogyi L, Chuttani R, Croffie J, et al. ASGE technology status evaluation report. Biliary and pancreatic stents. Gastrointest Endosc 2009;63:910–9.
2. Costamagna G, Gabbrielli A, Mutignani M, et al. Treatment of "obstructive" pain by endoscopic drainage in patients with pancreatic head carcinoma. Gastrointest Endosc 1993;39:774–7.
3. Tham TC, Lichtenstein DR, Vandervoort J, et al. Pancreatic duct stents for "obstructive type" pain in pancreatic malignancy. Am J Gastroenterol 2000;95: 956–60.
4. Freeman ML, DiSario JA, Nelson DB, et al. Risk factors for post-ERCP pancreatitis: a prospective, multicenter study. Gastrointest Endosc 2001;54:425–34.
5. Freeman ML, Nelso DB, Sherman S, et al. Complications of endoscopic biliary sphincterotomy. N Engl J Med 1996;335:909–18.

6. Loperfido S, Angelini G, Benedetti G, et al. Major early complications from diagnostic and therapeutic ERCP: a prospective multicenter study. Gastrointest Endosc 1998;48:1–10.

7. Masci E, Toti G, Mariani A, et al. Complications of diagnostic and therapeutic ERCP: a prospective multicenter study. Am J Gastroenterol 2001;96:417–23.

8. Dumonceau JM, Andriulli A, Devière J, et al. ESGE Guideline: prophylaxis of post-ERCP pancreatitis. Endoscopy 2010;42:503–15.

9. Elmunzer BJ, Waljee A, Elta G, et al. A meta-analysis of rectal NSAIDs in the prevention of post-ERCP pancreatitis. Gut 2008;57:1262–7.

10. Smithline A, Silverman W, Rogers D, et al. Effect of prophylactic main pancreatic duct stenting on the incidence of biliary endoscopic sphincterotomy-induced pancreatitis in high-risk patients. Gastrointest Endosc 1993;39:652–7.

11. Tarnasky PR, Palesch YY, Cunningham JT, et al. Pancreatic stenting prevents pancreatitis after biliary sphincterotomy in patients with sphincter of Oddi dysfunction. Gastroenterology 1998;115:1518–24.

12. Harewood GC, Pochron NL, Gostout CJ. Prospective, randomized controlled study of prophylactic pancreatic stent placement for endoscopic snare excision of duodenal papilla. Gastrointest Endosc 2005;62:367–70.

13. Andriulli A, Forlano R, Napolitano G, et al. Pancreatic duct stents in the prophylaxis of pancreatic damage after endoscopic retrograde cholangiopancreatography: a systemic analysis of benefits and associated risks. Digestion 2007;75:156–63.

14. Masci E, Mariani A, Curioni S, et al. Risk factors for pancreatitis following endoscopic retrograde cholangiopancreatography: a meta-analysis. Endoscopy 2003;35:830–4.

15. Singh P, Das A, Isenberg G, et al. Does prophylactic pancreatic stent placement reduce the risk of post-ERCP acute pancreatitis? A meta-analysis of controlled studies. Gastrointest Endosc 2004;60:544–50.

16. Mazaki T, Masuda H, Takayama T. Prophylactic pancreatic stent placement and post-ERCP pancreatitis: a systematic review and meta-analysis. Endoscopy 2010;42:842–52.

17. Freeman ML, Guda NM. Prevention of post-ERCP pancreatitis: a comprehensive review. Gastrointest Endosc 2004;59:845–63.

18. Kozarek RA. Pancreatic stents can induce ductal changes consistent with chronic pancreatitis. Gastrointest Endosc 1990;36:93–5.

19. Smith MT, Sherman S, Ikenberry SO, et al. Alterations in pancreatic ductal morphology following polyethylene pancreatic stent therapy. Gastrointest Endosc 1996;44:268–75.

20. Chahal P, Tarnasky P, Petersen B, et al. 5 Fr vs long 3 Fr pancreatic stents in patients at high risk for post-ERCP pancreatitis. Clin Gastroenterol Hepatol 2009;7:834–9.

21. Zolotarevsky E, Fehmi SM, Anderson MA, et al. Prophylactic 5 Fr pancreatic duct stents are superior to 3 Fr stents: a randomized controlled trial. Endoscopy 2011;43:325–30.

22. Maeda S, Hayashi H, Hosokawa O, et al. Prospective randomized pilot trial of selective biliary cannulation using pancreatic guide wire placement. Endoscopy 2003;35:721–4.

23. Brackbill S, Young S, Schoenfeld P, et al. A survey of physician practice on prophylactic pancreatic stents. Gastrointest Endosc 2006;64:45–52.

24. Dumonceau JM, Rigaux J, Kahaleh M, et al. Prophylaxis of post-ERCP pancreatitis: a practice survey. Gastrointest Endosc 2010;71:934–9.

25. Delhaye M, Arvanitakis M, Bali M, et al. Endoscopic therapy for chronic pancreatitis. Scand J Surg 2005;94:143–53.
26. Costamagna G, Bulajic M, Tringali A, et al. Multiple stenting of refractory pancreatic duct strictures in severe chronic pancreatitis: long-term results. Endoscopy 2006;38:254–9.
27. Cremer M, Devière J, Delhaye M, et al. Stenting in severe chronic pancreatitis: results of medium-term follow-up in seventy-six patients. Endoscopy 1991;23: 171–6.
28. Ponchon T, Bory RM, Hedelius F, et al. Endoscopic stenting for pain relief in chronic pancreatitis: results of a standardized protocol. Gastrointest Endosc 1995;42:452–6.
29. Eleftheriadis N, Dinu F, Delhaye M, et al. Long-term outcome after pancreatic stenting in severe chronic pancreatitis. Endoscopy 2005;37:223–30.
30. Dite P, Ruzicka M, Zboril V, et al. A prospective, randomized trial comparing endoscopic and surgical therapy for chronic pancreatitis. Endoscopy 2003;35: 553–8.
31. Cahen DL, Gouma DJ, Nio Y, et al. Endoscopic versus surgical drainage of the pancreatic duct in chronic pancreatitis. N Engl J Med 2007;356:676–84.
32. Rosch T, Daniel S, Scholz M, et al. Endoscopic treatment of chronic pancreatitis: a multicenter study of 1000 patients with long-term follow-up. Endoscopy 2002; 34:765–71.
33. Devière J, Bell RH Jr, Beger HG, et al. Treatment of chronic pancreatitis with endotherapy or surgery: critical review of randomized control trials. J Gastrointest Surg 2008;12:640–4.
34. Binmoeller KF, Jue P, Seifert H, et al. Endoscopic pancreatic stent drainage in chronic pancreatitis and a dominant stricture: long-term results. Endoscopy 1995;27:638–44.
35. Farnbacher MJ, Mühldorfer S, Wehler M, et al. Interventional endoscopic therapy in chronic pancreatitis including temporary stenting: a definitive treatment? Scand J Gastroenterol 2006;41:111–7.
36. Smits ME, Badiga SM, Rauws EA, et al. Long-term results of pancreatic stents in chronic pancreatitis. Gastrointest Endosc 1995;42:461–7.
37. Ishihara T, Yamaguchi T, Seza K, et al. Efficacy of s-type stents for the treatment of the main pancreatic duct stricture in patients with chronic pancreatitis. Scand J Gastroenterol 2006;41:744–50.
38. Boursier J, Quentin V, Le Tallec V, et al. Endoscopic treatment of painful chronic pancreatitis: evaluation of a new flexible multiperforated plastic stent. Gastroenterol Clin Biol 2008;32:801–5.
39. Raju GS, Gomez G, Xiao SY, et al. Effect of a novel pancreatic stent design on short-term pancreatic injury in a canine model. Endoscopy 2006;38:260–5.
40. Kozarek RA, Ball TJ, Patterson DJ, et al. Endoscopic transpapillary therapy for disrupted pancreatic duct and peripancreatic fluid collections. Gastroenterology 1991;100:1362–70.
41. Devière J, Bueso H, Baize M, et al. Complete disruption of the main pancreatic duct: endoscopic management. Gastrointest Endosc 1995;42:445–51.
42. Moon SH, Kim MH, Park do H, et al. Modified fully covered self expandable metal stents with antimigration features for benign pancreatic duct strictures in advance chronic pancreatitis with a focus on the safety profile and reducing migration. Gastrointest Endosc 2010;72:86–91.
43. Eisendrath P, Devière J. Expandable metal stents for benign pancreatic duct obstruction. Gastrointest Endosc Clin N Am 1999;9:547–54.

44. Hookey LC, Debroux S, Delhaye M, et al. Endoscopic drainage of pancreatic-fluid collections in 116 patients: a comparison of etiologies, drainage techniques, and outcomes. Gastrointest Endosc 2006;63:635–43.

45. Baron TH, Harewood GC, Morgan DE, et al. Outcome differences after endoscopic drainage of pancreatic necrosis, acute pancreatic pseudocysts, and chronic pancreatic pseudocysts. Gastrointest Endosc 2002;56:7–17.

46. Giovannini M, Pesenti C, Rolland AL, et al. Endoscopic ultrasound-guided drainage of pancreatic pseudocyst or pancreatic abscesses using a therapeutic echo endoscope. Endoscopy 2001;33:473–7.

47. Varadajulu S, Trevino J, Wilcox CM, et al. Randomized trial comparing EUS and surgery for pancreatic pseudocyst drainage. Gastrointest Endosc 2010;71: AB116.

48. Arvanitakis M, Delhaye M, Bali MA, et al. Pancreatic fluid collections: a randomized controlled trial regarding stent removal after endoscopic transmural drainage. Gastrointest Endosc 2007;65:609–19.

49. Cahen D, Rauws E, Fockens P, et al. Endoscopic drainage of pancreatic pseudocysts: long-term outcome and procedural factors associated with safe and successful treatment. Endoscopy 2005;37:977–83.

50. Lawrence C, Howell DA, Stefan AM, et al. Disconnected pancreatic tail syndrome: potential for endoscopic therapy and results of long-term follow-up. Gastrointest Endosc 2008;67:673–9.

51. Devière J, Antaki F. Disconnected pancreatic tail syndrome: a plea for multidisciplinarity. Gastrointest Endosc 2008;67:680–2.

52. Arvanitakis M, Delhaye M, Bali MA, et al. Endoscopic treatment of external pancreatic fistulas: when draining the main pancreatic duct is not enough. Am J Gastroenterol 2007;102:516–24.

53. Tessier G, Bories E, Arvanitakis M, et al. EUS-guided pancreatogastrostomy and pancreatobulbostomy for the treatment of pain in patients with pancreatic ductal dilatation inaccessible for transpapillary endoscopic therapy. Gastrointest Endosc 2007;65:233–41.

54. Kahaleh M, Hermandez AJ, Tokar J, et al. EUS-guided pancreaticogastrostomy: analysis of its efficacy to drain inaccessible pancreatic ducts. Gastrointest Endosc 2007;65:224–30.

55. Pai CG, Suvarna D, Bhat G. Endoscopic treatment as first-line therapy for pancreatic ascites and pleural effusion. J Gastroenterol Hepatol 2009;24(7):1198–202.

56. Rogers SJ, Cello JP, Schecter WP. Endoscopic retrograde cholangiopancreatography in patients with pancreatic trauma. J Trauma 2010;68(3):538–44.

57. Bhasin DK, Rana SS, Rawal P. Endoscopic retrograde pancreatography in pancreatic trauma: need to break the mental barrier. J Gastroenterol Hepatol 2009;24(5):720–8.

58. Abe N, Sugiyama M, Suzuki Y, et al. Preoperative endoscopic pancreatic stenting for prophylaxis of pancreatic fistula development after distal pancreatectomy. Am J Surg 2006;191(2):198–200.

59. Rieder B, Krampulz D, Adolf J, et al. Endoscopic pancreatic sphincterotomy and stenting for preoperative prophylaxis of pancreatic fistula after distal pancreatectomy. Gastrointest Endosc 2010;72(3):536–42.

60. Baron TH, Kozarek R, Carr-Locke DL. ERCP. Philadelphia: Saunders Elsevier; 2008. Chapter 16.

Expandable Metal Stents for Malignant Colorectal Strictures

Alessandro Repici, MD*, Daniel de Paula Pessoa Ferreira, MD

KEYWORDS

- Large-bowel obstruction • Self-expanding metallic stents
- Placement • Outcome

Malignant large-bowel obstruction can present as a life-threatening medical and surgical condition. The role of endoscopic management of this condition has significantly changed in the last 15 years. In the early 1990s luminal recanalization by laser debulking was the only available endoscopic option with high success rates in the treatment of primary malignant colonic obstruction.[1] In the largest retrospective study of 272 patients treated with a neodymium-yttrium aluminum garnet laser for obstructing rectosigmoid tumors, successful relief of the obstruction was achieved in 85% of patients.[2] Unfortunately, this technique was challenging to apply in patients with acute clinical obstruction, and required several sessions to successfully relieve the obstruction, with large mass lesions being less likely to respond to treatment.[2]

Lelcuk and colleagues[3] first described colon decompression by transanal insertion of a nasogastric tube in 1986. In 1991, Dohmoto and colleagues[4] pioneered the placement of the first expandable metal stent for palliation of malignant rectal obstruction. Subsequently Spinelli and colleagues[5] reported palliation of left-sided colonic strictures in a series of patients treated by placement of a modified Gianturco-Rosch stent. Several years later, Tejero and colleagues[6] were the first to report 2 cases of colonic stent placement preoperatively to allow elective surgery. Since those preliminary experiences, successful management of malignant large-bowel obstruction using self-expanding metallic stents (SEMS) has been increasingly reported by several groups of investigators.[7–10] With the introduction of dedicated enteral stents, this technique has gained more popularity and has been progressively incorporated in clinical practice, thus becoming the most effective alternative to surgery in management of patients with malignant large-bowel obstruction.[11–14]

Digestive Endoscopy Unit, IRCCS Istituto Clinico Humanitas, Via Manzoni 56, 20089 Rozzano, Milano, Italy
* Corresponding author.
E-mail address: alessandro.repici@humanitas.it

Gastrointest Endoscopy Clin N Am 21 (2011) 511–533
doi:10.1016/j.giec.2011.04.005
1052-5157/11/$ – see front matter © 2011 Elsevier Inc. All rights reserved.

SURGERY FOR MALIGNANT LARGE-BOWEL OBSTRUCTION

Malignant obstruction is the most common cause of emergency colorectal surgery.[11,15] Among patients with primary colorectal cancer, 15% to 20% present with obstructive symptoms.[16–19]

Most patients presenting with obstructive colorectal cancer have advanced stage disease, are often elderly, and are overall in poor medical condition. All of these factors adversely affect the operative risk, prognosis, and mortality. In addition, emergent surgery in a patient with an unprepared colon leads to significant morbidity and mortality.[19] To date, there is no consensus regarding the optimal surgical approach for the management of patients seen on an emergency basis with obstruction from colorectal cancer.

In the past, the standard treatment of malignant left-sided colonic obstruction was a 3-stage approach that involved creation of a colostomy to relieve the obstruction, followed by a second surgery to resect the tumor, and then a third one for colostomy closure. Unfortunately, this approach resulted in a prolonged hospital stay and worse long-term prognosis and thus has been almost completely abandoned. During the 1970s, a 2-stage approach with primary resection of tumor, closure of the rectal stump, and proximal-end colostomy (Hartmann procedure) became increasingly popular. Still, mortality and morbidity figures for emergency surgical decompression remained high, up to 10% and 60%, respectively.[20–22] Furthermore, reversal of the colostomy was not possible in 40%–60% of patients because of advanced disease or the presence of significant comorbid conditions.[20–22] It is well known that a stoma itself can have a profound adverse effect on the quality of life of these patients. Therefore, it is not surprising that, in recent years, 1-stage surgical procedures, with and without intraoperative colonic lavage have been advocated in selected patients as an alternative to a Hartmann procedure. Although 1-stage resection and anastomosis is considered to be a better option than primary resection with end colostomy in left-sided colonic obstruction, this is not true for all patients. Several important predictors of outcome in patients with large-bowel obstruction caused by colorectal cancer have been identified and can be used to decide the best surgical approach. These include age, American Society of Anesthesiologists (ASA) score, operative urgency, and Dukes stage.[22,23] Based on these factors it would be more appropriate to choose a simpler and safer procedure such as the Hartmann operation or even a diverting colostomy for patients deemed to be at high risk. This approach was reflected in a 2001 survey of American gastrointestinal surgeons. Sixty-seven percent would perform a Hartmann operation and 26% a simple colostomy in high-risk patients.[24] Moreover, even in good operative candidates, only 53% of gastrointestinal surgeons would perform a resection with primary anastomosis. The surgical subspecialty and experience seems to be a primary factor in the choice of operation and its final outcome. It has been shown that a primary anastomosis is more likely to be performed by colorectal consultants than general surgeons, and consultants generally than unsupervised trainees.[25]

In a study by The Association of Coloproctology of Great Britain and Ireland (ACPGBI) the mortality after surgery was similar between ACPGBI and non-ACPGBI members,[26] although the data submitted were voluntary. The Large Bowel Cancer Project showed that registrars had a higher mortality rate than consultants after primary resection for obstruction in the late 1970s, and this did not changed 20 years later.[25] Other studies have clearly shown that surgery by unsupervised trainees has significantly greater morbidity, mortality, and anastomotic dehiscence rates.[27]

Given these considerations, the use of colorectal stents to manage patients with acute bowel obstruction has became popular and gained acceptance even by the surgical community who consider the endoscopic approach to be a safe and viable approach in an attempt toward a safer and more effective surgical resection of obstructing neoplasia.[28]

INDICATIONS FOR COLORECTAL STENTING

Acute large-bowel obstruction caused by colorectal cancer is a common major surgical emergency, usually afflicting the left colon. If untreated, bowel obstruction causes rapid distension of enteral loops with a progression from abdominal pain, nausea, and vomiting to ischemia, bowel rupture, sepsis, and eventual death. In this setting, the use of SEMS has been proposed to provide a persisting opening of the neoplastic stricture and relieve acute obstruction. Indications for colorectal stent placement should be defined after a thorough evaluation of baseline clinical and radiologic data, with a multidisciplinary team of radiologists, surgeons, and endoscopists. Considerations for stent placement include the patient's laboratory examination, medical history, and imaging studies in conjunction with the individual scenario. Images from a thin-section computed tomography (CT) scan with multiplanar reformatted reconstructions (**Fig. 1**) can allow accurate delineation of relevant anatomy and morphology of the obstruction, as well as detection of any extraluminal spread or metastasis of the disease.

Once the evaluation is completed, the 2 main indications for colonic stenting in malignant colorectal obstruction are: (1) preoperative colonic decompression before colonic resection, the so-called bridge to surgery and (2) palliation of obstructing tumors not suitable for curative surgical resection.

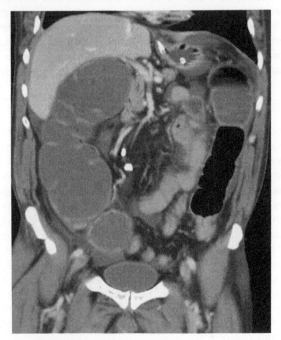

Fig. 1. CT scan showing distended bowel loops and obstruction at the level of the descending colon.

SEMS placement allows colonic decompression with relief of acute obstruction, stabilization of the acute illness, preoperative bowel preparation, and preoperative colonoscopy to assess for synchronous cancers. If definitive surgery is indicated, patients may then undergo a 1-stage surgical procedure, even with a laparoscopic approach, with a primary anastomosis in a more elective setting and a better-prepared patient.

However, in the presence of metastatic disease or in patients with prohibitive operative risk, endoscopic decompression with stent placement may become the definitive palliative procedure.

Absolute contraindications to colorectal stenting are: (1) perforation documented with free intraperitoneal gas, (2) very distal rectal lesions with a healthy margin of tissue less than 3 to 4 cm from the anal sphincter, and (3) peritoneal carcinomatosis.[29] Uncorrectable coagulopathy is a relative contraindication for SEMS placement, and in case of prolonged bleeding times, stenting can be performed after administration of fresh frozen plasma and platelets, as necessary.

Colonic obstruction may also arise from advanced extracolonic malignancy, including metastatic gynecologic, pancreatic, bladder, prostatic or small-bowel tumors. In these cases, extrinsic compression or invasion into the colon may lead to partial or complete obstruction of the lumen. In contrast to primary colonic cancer, these patients often have complex stricturing of the gut, potentially at more than 1 location, related to the underlying malignancy. They may also have underlying adhesions from previous debulking surgery and/or chemoradiotherapy. The combination of these multiple factors, including radiation therapy and peritoneal carcinomatosis, which can result in bowel immobilization, may contribute to decreased success and increased complication rate of colon stent placement in patients with extracolonic malignancies.[30,31] Therefore it seems to be reasonable that endoscopic placement of a colon stent in this setting should only be undertaken in a limited subgroup of patients in whom either decompressive surgery is not feasible or alternative therapies have already failed. Patients and their family members should be made aware of the lower success rate and the potential for serious complications before attempting stent placement for a bowel obstruction caused by extracolonic malignancies.

COLORECTAL STENTS

The early experience of colorectal stent placement involved use of stents designed for other locations, such as esophageal stents (**Fig. 2**). In 1998 a prototype nitinol stent specifically designed for colonic lesions was developed and tested in a prospective trial by the Leuven group.[32] In the following years, many stents have been designed specifically for use in the lower gastrointestinal tract and are available in a variety of lengths and diameters, so that the appropriate stent can be selected based on factors such as the length of the obstructed section of bowel and anatomic location of the obstruction. Various SEMS are composed of metals such as stainless steel, Elgiloy, or nitinol and may be uncovered or covered with a polyurethane, polyethylene, or silicone coating to resist tumor ingrowth and tissue hyperplasia. Stainless steel and Elgiloy stents have been almost completely abandoned and replaced by nitinol stents, which are nonferromagnetic and are magnetic resonance imaging compatible.[33] Nonetheless, they may produce imaging artifacts such as mild local field inhomogeneities on magnetic resonance imaging and beam-hardening on CT depending on stent shape and alloy composition.[34,35]

A recent study has shown that CT colonography may be used safely for preoperative examination of the proximal colon after metallic stent placement in patients with

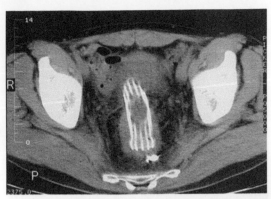

Fig. 2. CT scan image of an esophageal Ultraflex stent placed across a malignant rectal stricture.

acute colon obstruction caused by cancer.[36] According to the size of the stent deployment system, 2 different classes of stents can be distinguished: the so-called TTS (through the scope), which is mounted on a small size catheter that can pass through an endoscope with a working channel of at least 3.7 mm (**Fig. 3**); and the so-called OTW or (over the wire), which is mounted on a larger delivery system and cannot pass through the working channel of the endoscope (**Fig. 4**). With the development of very flexible nitinol SEMS (**Fig. 5**) mounted on a small diameter delivery system that can pass through the working channel of an adult colonoscope, therapeutic gastroscope, or duodenoscope, almost all intestinal obstructions that are within the reach of an endoscope are amenable to endoscopic decompression, including those in the ascending colon. Theoretically, the larger diameter stents are better suited to accommodate solid stool in the left colon and according to a recent study a larger diameter stent is not associated with an increased risk of complications even in patients undergoing chemotherapy.[37] US Food and Drug Administration (FDA) approved and CE marked (Conformité Européene, available for European market) colorectal stents are listed in **Table 1**.

Available studies comparing the performance of different stents suggest that there is no clear-cut advantage in the use of covered SEMS compared with uncovered

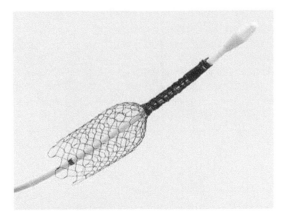

Fig. 3. Over the wire (OTW) Ultraflex Precision stent partially expanded over its 16 Fr catheter. (*Courtesy of* Boston Scientific Corp, Inc; with permission.)

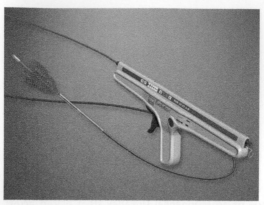

Fig. 4. Through-the-scope (TTS) Evolution stent (Cook Endoscopy). Release is controlled with a dedicated gun system. (*Courtesy of* Cook Endoscopy, Inc; with permission.)

SEMS in patients with malignant colonic obstruction either in the preoperative or palliative setting.[38] An uncovered stent provides adequate and effective decompression when placed as a bridge to surgery and when resection is performed within a short period of time after placement. When used for definitive palliation, covered stents might have the potential advantage of preventing tumor ingrowth and reobstruction thus reducing the need for further intervention. However, comparative studies and retrospective analysis of published data seem to indicate that this potential advantage is offset by the tendency of covered stents to migrate more commonly.[38–40] In an older study of 20 patients who presented with malignant colonic obstruction, 8 had SEMS placed for palliative decompression. Four patients had covered stents, all of which migrated within 3 to 4 days.[41] The other 4 patients had partially covered stents, and these remained patent and in place until the time of death. In another nonrandomized study, 33 patients underwent successful SEMS placement for definitive palliation of malignant colonic obstruction. Three types of stents were used: fully covered, partially covered, and uncovered. Stent migration occurred in 11 of 33 patients (33%), none of which were uncovered.[39]

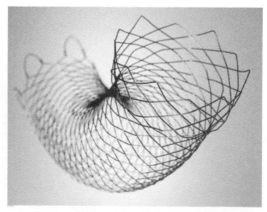

Fig. 5. The Wallflex colonic stent (Boston Scientific). (*Courtesy of* Boston Scientific Corp, Inc; with permission.)

Table 1
Overview of commercially available stents in the Unites States and elsewhere

Stent Colonic	Manufacturer	Expanded Length (mm)	Diameter (mm)	TTS/OTW	Introduction System Fr Size	Working Length (cm)
Evolution colonic stent	Cook Medical	60, 80, 100	30, 25	TTS	10	230
Ultraflex Precision colonic stent[a]	Boston Scientific/Microvasive, Natick, MA, USA	57, 87, 117	30, 25	OTW	16	105
Wallstent[a] colonic and duodenal endoprosthesis	Boston Scientific/Microvasive, Natick, MA, USA	60, 90	18, 20, 22	TTS	10	135
WallFlex[a] colonic stent	Boston Scientific/Microvasive, Natick, MA, USA	60, 90, 120	30, 25 27, 22	TTS	10	135 230
Colonic Z-Stent[a]	Cook Medical, Winston-Salem, NC, USA	40, 60, 80, 100, 120	35, 25	OTW	31	40
Silky colorectal stent	Stentech, Seoul, South Korea	Covered/uncovered 50, 60, 70; 80, 90, 100, 120, 140, 160	30	TTS	10	70 80
Niti-S colorectal stent	Taewoong Medical Co, Ltd, Seoul, South Korea	Uncovered 60, 80, 100	28, 20 30, 22 30, 24 28, 20	OTW	16 18	70 150
Niti-S colorectal stent	Taewoong Medical Co, Ltd, Seoul, South Korea	Covered 60, 80, 100	30, 22 30, 24	OTW	20 22	70 150
Bonastent colorectal stent	Standard Sci.Tech Inc	Uncovered 60, 80, 100	22, 24, 26	TTS / OTW	10 12	140 230
Bonastent colorectal stent	Standard Sci.Tech Inc	Covered 60, 80, 100 30/50/80	22, 24, 26	TTS / OTW	10 12	140 230
Hanaro colorectal stent	M.I TECH Co Ltd	40, 70, 100	22	TTS	10.5	210
ECO stent	Leufen Medizintechnik OHG	Uncovered 80, 100	30, 36	OTW	24	70 110
SX-ELLA stent colorectal	ELLA-CS, Prague, Czech Republic	82, 90, 113, 135 75, 88, 112, 123, 136	20, 25, 30	OTW	13	95
Micro-Tech colon and rectum stent	Micro-tech Europe, Dusseldorf, Germany	Uncovered 80, 100, 120 Covered 80, 100, 120 50, 70, 90	30, 36 25, 30	TTS	10, 24	110, 230

[a] FDA approved.

In a pooled analysis of colonic SEMS by Sebastian and colleagues[38] that included 54 studies, 170 covered SEMS were placed and 52 (30.5%) were reported to migrate on subsequent follow-up.

More recently, Lee and colleagues[42] reported their experience comparing uncovered and covered SEMS in 80 patients with malignant colonic obstruction. The investigators used SEMS made of a mesh of single-strand wire of a nickel-titanium alloy (Niti-S, Colon TTS; Taewoong Medical Co, Seoul, South Korea). The uncovered stents were cylindrical, but the covered stents had a dumbbell shape with flange ends that were partially covered with a polyurethane membrane. In the covered stent group, there were 9 late complications, including 6 episodes of stent migration, 1 reported tumor overgrowth, and 2 cases of stool impaction. Tumor ingrowth was reported in only 3 patients in the uncovered stent group thus confirming that there is no obvious advantage in using covered stents compared with uncovered stents in the treatment of patients with malignant colonic obstruction either in the preoperative or palliative setting.

The increased risk of migration of covered stents in colorectal strictures could be mainly related to local factors, inherent to the colon's anatomy, including its wide caliber and motility, which may facilitate stent migration. The lower risk of migration of uncovered stents is because these stents progressively incorporate deeply into the wall of the tumor and surrounding tissues by pressure necrosis, firmly anchoring the stent.[37–39]

PLACEMENT TECHNIQUES

Since its original description by Dohmoto and colleagues[4] in the early 1990s, the technique of preoperative colonic stenting has remained substantially unchanged in its general principles. Prophylactic antibiotics should be considered in patients with complete obstruction as the introduction of air may induce microperforation and bacteremia. Because patients who have complete obstruction usually have evacuated most feces below the lesion, colonic bowel preparation is unnecessary or even dangerous because it may promote worsening of the obstruction. The use of 1 or 2 generous cleansing enemas is usually suggested to improve endoscopic visibility in the segments below the stricture. If the stricture is located in the rectosigmoid the patient is placed in the supine position which favors radiologic definition of anatomic landmarks. If the stricture is located proximal to the sigmoid, the patient is initially placed in the left lateral position to better negotiate the left colon and afterwards turned to the supine position once the stricture has been reached with the endoscope.

In most cases, colorectal stenting is a well-tolerated procedure with minimal patient pain and discomfort especially if the lesion is located in the distal part of the colon. The use of moderate sedation with a combination of an opiate (eg, fentanyl) and a benzodiazepine (eg, midazolam) is commonly used.

From a technical standpoint, placement of an OTW stent differs in the final steps from placement of a TTS stent.

The OTW stents, because of their catheter length and diameter, are best reserved for those patients whose strictures are located in the rectum or in the distal part of the sigmoid within 20 to 30 cm from the anal verge. The advancement of the OTW stent catheter beyond this limit is challenging because the force to move the stent forward is applied outside the anus, far from the stricture and this normally causes looping of the catheter in the mobile sigmoid instead of a true advancement of the stent across the stricture. The technique of SEMS placement in the rectum and distal sigmoid using an OTW stent is analogous to esophageal stent placement.

First the scope is advanced until the anal (distal) end of the stricture is identified. If an adult or therapeutic endoscope can be easily passed through the lesion, the authors suggest that stent placement is not undertaken because of the high risk of migration. However, no data are available to support this recommendation, which is based on personal experience. Conversely, there are data that strongly discourage dilation of the stricture either before or after stent placement because this significantly increases the risk of colonic perforation.[43,44] A recent ex vivo experimental study on freshly excised human colon cancer specimens has confirmed that dilation of colorectal cancer strictures is associated with a high risk of perforation.[45] According to the results of this elegant study, histopathologic and morphologic factors that cause a decrease in the elastic compliance of the lumen correlated with perforation risk more than dilation parameters such as balloon pressure. The best predictor for perforation was a combination of severe stricture and pronounced proliferation of peritumoral collagen fibers. Annular growth and fewer residual smooth muscle cells in the muscularis propria exhibiting tumor encroachment were also associated with an increased risk. because these factors are not known at the time of placement. Perforation is quite unpredictable and can occur regardless of the type of dilation performed.

After reaching the stricture, a guidewire is gently advanced under fluoroscopic guidance across the stricture. Air insufflation usually creates a contrast effect that may help to define fluoroscopically the bowel anatomy beyond the stricture and allow tracking of guidewire advancement above the stricture. If this contrast effect is not well defined or if doubts remain about anatomy and/or stricture morphology, a water soluble (meglumine diatrizoate, Gastrografin) contrast medium can be injected through the working channel of the endoscope. In addition, a hydrophilic or hybrid biliary guidewire preloaded through a biliary double or triple lumen occlusion balloon or catheter is used to inject contrast and cannulate under endoscopic and fluoroscopic guidance as is done during endoscopic retrograde cholangiography (ERCP). Once the wire has passed through the stricture, the catheter is advanced over the guidewire as far as possible and the standard guidewire is exchanged for a stiffer one. In cases of high-grade obstructions or sharply angulated strictures or eccentric position of the residual lumen, it may be challenging to introduce the guidewire in the correct orientation and safely advance it through the strictures. In such a case the use of a sphincterotome, which can be rotated and the tip flexed, is extremely useful in negotiating the correct direction to allow advancement of the guidewire.[46] Alternatively, side-viewing endoscopes can also be used to allow access to sharply angulated strictures located at the distal sigmoid that cannot be approached with frontal view scope because of their eccentric position.[47]

The length of the stent chosen should be about 4 to 6 cm longer than the estimated length of the stricture to allow an adequate margin of stent on either side of the obstruction.[48]

At this point if an OTW stent is used, the scope is withdrawn leaving the guide wire in place well above the stricture. The endoscope is reinserted alongside the guide wire to monitor (together with fluoroscopy) the advancement of the predeployed stent and to precisely position the distal end during deployment. If a TTS stent is chosen, the stent is advanced through the working channel of the endoscope across the stricture (**Fig. 6**) and then deployed under fluoroscopic and endoscopic guidance. During TTS stent deployment the physician handling the endoscope should gently but firmly pull back the external catheter of the stent to balance the tendency of the stent to move forward (away from the tip of the endoscope) because of advancement of the internal pushing catheter. Most TTS stents have a point of no return marker on the external portion of

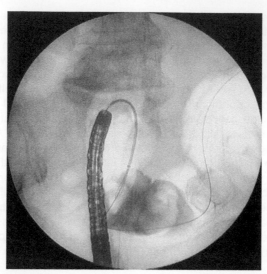

Fig. 6. TTS stent is advanced across the stricture over a guidewire positioned well beyond the target lesion.

the delivery catheter that correlates with a radiologic marker on the constraining sheath at the level of the stent, indicating the point at which the stent cannot be reconstrained in case of improper positioning. Once the stent is deployed fully, the ends of the stent should be inspected carefully by fluoroscopy and contrast injected into the stent to assess complete patency and exclude perforation. Definition of technical success includes correct opening of the stent across the stricture with passage of fecal material and absence of perforation. The definition of clinical success varies, but is most frequently colonic decompression with resolution of obstructive symptoms within 72 hours of stent placement.[14]

In most cases, reports and studies on colonic SEMS have come from tertiary referral hospitals and colorectal stenting is still considered a technically demanding and challenging endoscopic procedure. However, patients with obstructive colorectal cancer can present in the emergency departments of community or district general hospitals. These patients may be too ill to be transferred to tertiary referral centers for colonic stenting. The retrospective study of Garcia-Cano and colleagues,[49] has shown the reproducibility of colonic stenting for malignant colorectal obstruction in both community/district general hospitals and tertiary centers with high success rates. They reported 175 attempts to insert colorectal SEMS, with 19 (8.6%) strictures proximal to the left colon. Technical success was achieved in 93% and clinical success in 85%. Stents served as a bridge to surgery in 41% and as definitive palliation in 38%. Perforation occurred in 4%, with death in 1%. The investigators concluded that colonic stent placement can be feasibly performed in general endoscopic practice.

OUTCOME FOLLOWING COLONIC SEMS PLACEMENT

Twenty years from its introduction into clinical practice, colonic stenting has evolved from an experimental therapy performed with nondedicated devices to an accepted alternative method for palliation of inoperable colorectal cancer and for preoperative minimally invasive endoscopic decompression of obstructed patients with operable disease, so-called bridge to surgery. The outcome following these 2 different indications are discussed separately because both have specific peculiarities and have been evaluated in dedicated clinical studies. Median technical success rates, which are not strictly related to stent indication, are achieved in 96.2%, ranging from 66.6% to 100%.[14,29,38] The median rate of clinical success in a recent systematic review was 92%, ranging from 46% to 100% with extremely variable definitions of clinical success among more than 80 different studies evaluated.[14]

Palliation

Despite improvement in early detection of colorectal cancer, patients presenting with clinical obstruction at diagnosis still range between 7% and 29%.[28,50] Neoplastic strictures located distal to the splenic flexure represent 78% of all cases. Unfortunately, up to 19% of such patients already have distant metastases at diagnosis, and two-thirds of those are considered unsuitable for curative surgery.[45,46]

The management strategy for patients with locally advanced disease and/or distant metastasis presenting with obstruction is complex. On the one hand assuring patency of the bowel lumen and recovering bowel transit is an absolute clinical priority; on the other hand, prognosis of disease determines the aggressiveness of treatment.

Both synchronous metastasis and bowel obstruction are considered poor prognostic factors as well as high preoperative levels of carcinoembryonic antigen, histologic grade, extension of liver metastasis, or peritoneal metastases.[51-54]

The use of colonic stenting for palliation of patients with locally advanced or metastatic disease has been extensively investigated. Three randomized controlled trials (RCTs) comparing colostomy versus SEMS for palliation of malignant colonic obstruction have been reported in the last several years. The first study was published in 2004 by Xinopulos and colleagues,[9] who randomized 30 patients. Stent placement was achieved in 93.3% (14/15 patients) with no stent-related mortality reported.[9] In 57% (8/14) of patients in whom the stent was successfully placed, stenting provided long-term effective restoration of the luminal patency with no occlusive symptoms until death. Mean survival was 21.4 months in the SEMS group and 20.9 months in the colostomy group. Mean hospital stay was quite high in both groups and significantly higher in patients receiving colostomy (28 days vs 60 days). However, the small sample size of the study and some intrinsic limitations in study design might have limited the ability to detect differences between groups.

In the same year, Fiori and colleagues[55] published another small series in which 22 patients were randomized to either colostomy or SEMS. Mortality was 0% in both groups and morbidity was not significantly different. The advantage seen in the stent group was a shorter time to resumption of oral intake and restoration of bowel function, and a reduced hospital stay. This study was limited by the small simple size and lack of consistent follow-up.

The Dutch Stent-in I multicenter RCT was planned to randomize patients with incurable colorectal cancer to SEMS or surgery. The study was terminated prematurely after enrolling 21 patients because of a high rate of stent-related perforations resulting in 3 deaths among 10 patients in the SEMS group.[56,57] There is no clear explanation for such a high perforation rate; the investigators pointed out that limited safety data existed for the stent used (WallFlex, Boston Scientific Natick, MA). Several previous and subsequent studies using the same WallFlex stent for colonic obstruction for palliative management have described a perforation rate of about 5%[12,58-60] which is much lower that the Dutch study and in line with what is commonly observed with other stents.

The findings of a few prospective trials and many recent retrospective series further demonstrate the usefulness of SEMS for definitive palliative treatment of malignant colorectal strictures.[61–69] SEMS can provide rapid and effective relief of obstructive symptoms, with acceptable morbidity and need for reintervention and extremely low mortality. The SEMS placement procedure, typically performed with the patient under moderate sedation, entails less acute debilitation, more rapid recovery, and a shorter hospital stay compared with surgical alternatives. Such benefits are of particular value in obstructed patients with limited life expectancy when surgical treatment may be considered even unethical and with significant implications for the quality of life.[70]

A recent retrospective comparison of outcome between stenting (71 patients) and surgery (73 patients) has shown SEMS to be not only an effective and acceptable therapy for initial palliation of malignant colorectal obstruction but also showed long-term efficacy comparable with that of surgery.[71] Although the patency duration of the initially placed stent was shorter than that of surgery, placement of a second stent within the first stent when reobstruction occurred prolonged the benefit of endo-scopically treated patients and the median bowel patency was comparable with that of the surgical group. Data on the long-term efficacy of stenting for palliation has recently been confirmed in a large retrospective study; a long-term clinical success rate was achieved in 77.2% with a mean in situ period of 128 days and stent patency until death was achieved in 88.5% of patients.[44] A retrospective claims analysis of the Medicare Provider Analysis and Review (MedPAR) data set has been conducted to identify inpatient hospitalizations for colostomy or stent placement for the treatment of colon cancer with the aim of comparing economic outcomes.[72] Using the Medicare Cost Report, hospitalization costs were derived by applying the cost-to-charge ratio to the reported charges in MedPAR. Compared with colostomy, the median hospital stay (8 vs 12 days; $P<.0001$) and the median cost ($15,071 vs $24,695; $P<.001$) per claim were significantly less for stent placement. The study concluded that, although the technical and clinical outcomes for colostomy and stent placement appeared compa-rable, stent placement was less costly and associated with shorter hospital stay and fewer complications.

Quality of life and symptom control in patients with colonic strictures caused by advanced incurable disease (both colonic and extracolonic malignancies) were eval-uated in a prospective study including 44 patients treated with SEMS placement (30 patients) or surgical diversion (14 patients).[73] All patients were evaluated with vali-dated quality-of-life scores used for colorectal cancer (the Colon Symptoms score and the Functional Assessment of Cancer Therapy - Colorectal [FACT-C] score). Both SEMS placement and surgical diversion provided durable improvement in symp-toms of large-bowel obstruction. Stent placement was associated with improved overall quality-of-life scores and gastrointestinal symptom-specific quality-of-life scores. As the study progressed, fewer patients were willing to consider surgical diversion as referring physicians and patients became more familiar with SEMS.

Bridge to Surgery

It is well recognized from the surgical literature that mortality and morbidity rates are significantly higher for colorectal surgery in an emergency situation in contrast to an elective operation.[26–28] In patients with malignant colonic obstruction who are candi-dates for surgical resection, placement of a colonic SEMS allows colonic decompres-sion (**Fig. 7**A, B) without the morbidity and mortality of urgent surgery.[14,38] SEMS placement seems to result in significantly lower complication rates, shorter hospital stays, higher rates of primary anastomosis, and lower rates of colostomy compared with urgent surgery. Mortality with SEMS placement is similar to that with urgent

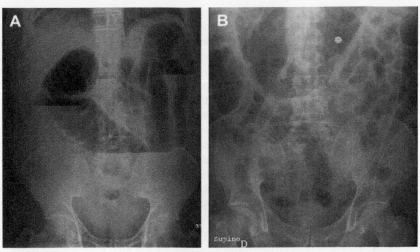

Fig. 7. (*A*) Fluoroscopic image of an acute obstruction caused by a sigmoid cancer. (*B*) The same patient after successful stent placement.

surgery, and the complication rate is usually less than 5%.[29] Moreover, the relief of symptoms provided by SEMS placement allows additional time to stabilize the patient, address underlying comorbid medical illnesses, perform a thorough staging evaluation of the cancer (including complete colonoscopy), and offers the opportunity to provide neoadjuvant therapy in patients with rectal cancer. In this way, colorectal stent placement serves as a favorable bridge to surgery.

The advantage of relieving acute obstruction may be seen because patients can undergo laparoscopic resection after successful stent placement and decompression.

Morino and colleagues[74] first presented data on a small series of patients treated by SEMS placement for decompression of malignant obstruction followed by laparoscopic 1-stage resection. The investigators concluded that the strategy of SEMS placement followed by laparoscopic 1-stage resection resulted in good patient comfort, rapid postoperative recovery, and short hospital stay. Studies in a larger cohort of patients confirmed that colonic stenting followed by laparoscopic resection can result in a safe and effective minimally invasive approach in the management of malignant bowel obstruction.[75,76] Two studies have compared the outcomes of SEMS followed by elective open surgery with those of emergency surgery without prior stenting and showed an increase in the proportion of patients who underwent successful primary anastomosis in the stented group, with a reduction in stoma formation.[77,78] In the pooled review by Sebastian and colleagues[38] of 54 uncontrolled series of SEMS placement, including palliative indications, SEMS was found to be a useful option to avoid colostomy and facilitate a 1-stage operation. More recently, a systematic review including 88 studies (15 of which were comparative)[14] and another larger systematic review[79] have suggested that SEMS insertion is a safe and effective strategy in patients with acute obstruction allowing resection to be performed in an elective setting. However, the small sample sizes of the published studies, which are predominately retrospective with substantial differences in treatments, have limited the validity of these findings. Three prospective randomized trials were published recently with completely different results.

Cheung and colleagues[80] published an RCT comparing an endolaparoscopic approach (24 patients) with conventional open surgery (24 patients). In patients who were randomized to the endolaparoscopic group, SEMS placement for colonic decompression was attempted within 24 to 30 hours of admission and an elective laparoscopic-assisted resection was performed within 2 weeks of SEMS placement. Patients who were randomized to the open surgery group underwent an emergency Hartman procedure or colectomy with intraoperative irrigation on the same day of admission. For the endolaparoscopic group, no stent-related complications occurred. In 4 patients, endoluminal stent placement failed because of failure to cannulate the obstruction. Self-expanding metal stents were successfully implanted in the remaining 20 patients with successful decompression yielding technical and clinical success rates of 83%. Patients in the endolaparoscopic group had a significantly lower incidence of anastomotic leak and wound infection. Moreover, significantly more patients in the endolaparoscopic group had a successful 1-stage operation performed (16 vs 9, $P = .04$). None of the patients in the endolaparoscopic group had a permanent stoma compared with 6 patients in the emergency open surgery group ($P = .03$).

A second randomized trial, including 9 French centers has been recently reported with results in contrast with those of the Cheung study. Among the 70 patients eligible for the study, 60 were randomized and included for the final analysis (30 patients in each group).[81]

Concerning the primary outcome, 17 patients in the surgery group sustained a stoma placement versus 13 patients in the SEMS group ($P = .30$). No statistically significant difference was noted concerning the secondary outcomes. Sixteen attempts at SEMS placement (53.3%) were technical failures. Two colonic perforations occurred among the 30 randomized patients and 1 perforation occurred among the nonrandomized patients, leading to premature closure of the study before the expected number of 80 patients was reached.

A further study, including 25 hospitals in the Netherlands, randomized patients with acute colonic obstruction to receive colonic stenting as a bridge to surgery or emergency surgery.[82] The study was prematurely closed because 2 successive interim analyses showed increased 30-day mortality in the colonic stenting group mainly as a consequence of a high rate of poststenting complications. The study confirmed that in Dutch cooperative studies,[56] the perforation rate is much higher than reported in the literature (13%, 6 out of 47 stented patients) with a lower technical success rate (70%, 33 out of 47 patients).

The conflicting results from studies from China and France (obtained during the same period, 2002–2006) and the premature closure of the Dutch study highlight the need for further evidence-based evaluation of stenting as a bridge to surgery in the setting of further randomized trials or at least a further systematic quantitative review.

To date, only a few studies have evaluated the effect of SEMS insertion compared with emergency surgery on a long-term prognosis in patients with potentially curable colorectal cancer.

Subclinical perforation may occur during stent insertion and it has been demonstrated that SEMS insertion may lead to tumor cells spilling into the peripheral circulation.[83] The impact of such events on long-term oncologic outcome is still unknown and deserves further investigation.

A Japanese abstract[84] reported no difference in 3-year survival between 44 patients treated with SEMS insertion followed by resection and 40 patients who had emergency surgery (48% vs 50%). An English study noted a 3-year survival rate of 80% in 10 patients who had SEMS insertion as a bridge to potentially curative resection compared with 74% in 15 patients who underwent emergency resection, after a mean follow-up of 21 months.[13] In a recent Korean study, the 5-year survival rate was 44% in 24 patients with stage II and III colonic cancer after SEMS placement as a bridge to surgery versus 87% in 240 patients who had elective surgery for nonobstructing left-sided colonic cancer.[50]

The cost-effectiveness of SEMS is another important issue to be evaluated because metal stents are expensive. It is believed that their cost may be offset by the shorter hospital stay and the lower rate of colostomy formation. Two decision analysis studies from the United States and Canada have calculated the cost-effectiveness of 2 competing strategies (stenting followed by elective surgery vs emergency primary resection).[85,86] Both analysis concluded that colonic stenting followed by elective surgery is significantly more effective and cost efficient than emergency surgery as a consequence of reduced complication rates and hospital stay. A small retrospective study from the United Kingdom in 1998 showed that palliative stenting compared with surgical decompression allows saving a mean of £1769, whereas the stenting as a bridge to elective resection versus emergency Hartman resection followed by elective reversal saved a mean of £685.[87] Similar results were obtained by a Swiss study showing that SEMS was 19.7% less costly than surgery.[88] Although stents seem to be cost-effective, results are difficult to compare because costs calculations vary significantly in different health care systems, costs differ for palliation and bridge to surgery, and the cost of stents is likely to decrease with time.

COMPLICATIONS OF COLORECTAL SEMS

Colorectal stenting is a relatively low-risk procedure with a mortality rate of less than 1%.[44,58,64,70] Complications are usually divided into early (within 30 days), including perforation, bleeding, and misplacement, and late, including mainly stent migration, reobstruction, tenesmus, and more rarely perforation.

Overall, one of the most common complications of stent placement is stent occlusion caused by tumor ingrowth or overgrowth. The likelihood of stent occlusion by tumor growth increases with the time elapsed after stent placement because of the natural tendency of neoplasms to invade local tissues[64] thus making this complication more frequent in the setting of palliation of malignant strictures. A systemic review of the published data from 302 patients reported in 29 case series showed a rate of stent occlusion of 16% (49/302) in patients with a stent inserted for palliation.[89] In a multicenter European study, using the Ultraflex Precision stent for patients with inoperable disease, at 6 months, the rate of clinical success was 81% based on Kaplan-Meier analysis and intention-to-treat analysis, and clinical success was maintained until death in 86% of the nonsurvivors.[64] In the past, tumor ingrowth was treated with laser ablation therapy, but more recently, insertion of an additional stent (**Fig. 8**A, B) is becoming the standard treatment of tumor ingrowth or overgrowth.[29] In a more recent study, stent occlusion because of tumor ingrowth or overgrowth occurred in 8 patients (15.4%) at a mean time of 127 days, and was treated in most cases with successful additional stenting.[90]

In a recent Korean study, factors associated with a favorable outcome in colonic stenting were identified. Patients with shorter length stents (<10 cm) had better outcomes than those with longer length stents (≥10 cm; $P = .008$), and patients with a distal colorectal obstruction had better outcomes than those with a proximal colorectal obstruction ($P = .015$).[69] Except for 1 patient, most who experienced stent occlusion were treated successfully with placement of an additional overlapping stent. In those patients treated with an additional stent, reocclusion did not develop until the end of the follow-up period or the death of patient, thus confirming the clinical value of restenting in patients experiencing first stent obstruction.[44,71]

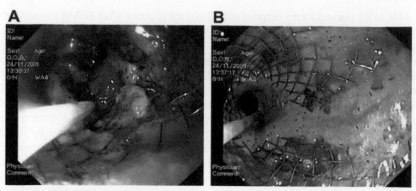

Fig. 8. (A) Endoscopic image of tumor ingrowth which led to reobstruction. (B) Same patient after insertion of a new stent within the original. Restoration of patency is confirmed by passage of fecal material through the stent lumen.

Stent migration may be asymptomatic or result in recurrence of obstructive symptoms or bleeding and/or tenesmus if the stent affects the anorectum. Removal of distally migrated stents from the rectum is not technically difficult and can often be performed manually without the use of an endoscope. The migration rates of uncovered stents range from 3% to 12%, whereas migration rates for covered stents are reported to be as high as 30% to 50%.[90]

Migration occurs more frequently after chemoradiotherapy because of tumor shrinkage, or in case of predeployment of laser debulking or balloon dilation.[29] Other factors that may predispose stent migration include placement within partially obstructed lesions, those caused by benign disease or extrinsic compression, use of inadequately sized stents,[91] and fecal impaction.[92] Stent migration occurs 3 times more frequently with stents placed in the distal rectum compared with the left colon.[93] As for stent obstruction, stent migration may be treated with the insertion of a second stent although there are no data on the outcome of restenting in this specific situation.

The complication considered most dangerous for the patient and most frightening for the physician is colonic perforation, which can occur at different stages of the procedure or after stent placement. Prestenting perforation (the so-called procedure-related perforation) accounts for 15% to 20% of cases and is usually related to wire or catheter misplacement or to stricture dilation, which is by now considered a well-known predisposing factor. Over distension of air in an already dilated proximal bowel may result in a closed-loop perforation away from the site of the lesion. Stent-related perforation may occur because of tumor fracture caused by the radial force of the stent or because of pressure of the stent ends on the healthy mucosa at the border of the tumor (**Fig. 9**). Overall, the risk of perforation has been estimated to be within 5%.[14,28,29,37,44] In some recent prospective trials, an unexpected high rate of perforation led to premature closure of the study.[56,81,82] A notable article on stent-related perforation that extensively reviewed studies of colorectal stenting from both English and foreign language publications[94] collected data on cause, timing, treatment, and mortality related to perforation. A total of 2287 patients from 82 articles were included in this analysis, which showed an overall perforation rate of 4.9%. Perforation rates for palliation and bridge to surgery were not significantly different (4.8% vs 5.4%, $P = .66$), with more than 80% of events occurring within 30 days of stent placement (half during or within 1 day of the procedure). Mortality related to perforation was 0.8% per stented patient, but the mortality of patients experiencing perforation was 16.2%. There was no

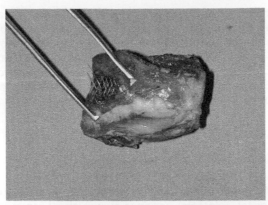

Fig. 9. Surgically resected specimen showing an enteral Wallstent. The sharp ends resulted in bowel perforation.

significant difference ($P = .78$) in mortality between the palliation and the bridge to surgery group. Concomitant chemotherapy, corticosteroid medications, and radiotherapy were significant risk factors for perforation. The overall perforation-related mortality was far less than that of patients undergoing emergency surgery for bowel obstruction. Bevacizumab-based chemotherapy is emerging as a major risk factor for poststenting perforation.[44] Several studies have found that bevacizumab therapy nearly triples the risk of perforation and significantly shortens the mean time to delayed perforation.[44,56,70,95] The antiangiogenic effect may weaken the bowel wall and might predispose to perforation at the point of SEMS pressure. This risk is probably independent from stenting itself because a recent review has clearly demonstrated that the addition of bevacizumab to cancer therapy significantly increases the risk of spontaneous gastrointestinal perforation compared with controls.[96]

The largest reported study of complications of SEMS from a single center with proven experience reveals several clinical predictors for complications.[44] Two of the most important risk factors, gender and degree of occlusion, were characteristics of the patients. Male gender increased susceptibility to an adverse event for unclear reasons. The completely occluded bowel may result in friable, microperforated tissue, and is associated with a severely tight stricture that makes SEMS deployment technically challenging. Other risk factors were related to procedural/endoscopic technique. The perforation rate was significantly lower when stents were placed by endoscopists experienced in pancreaticobiliary endoscopy. This is probably related to the basic skill set of endoscopists who perform therapeutic ERCP and who are familiar with guidewire manipulation, ability to traverse complex strictures, fluoroscopy images, and proper stent advancement and deployment.

SUMMARY

The surgical management of malignant colorectal obstruction is still controversial and has higher associated mortality and complication rates compared with elective surgery. SEMS placement has been proposed as an alternative therapeutic approach for colonic decompression of patients with acute malignant obstruction. SEMS placement may be used both as a bridge to surgery in patients who are good candidates for curative resection and for palliation of those patients presenting with advanced stage disease or with severe comorbid medical illnesses. Although data from recently published randomized clinical studies are conflicting, the role for preoperative stenting in the management of acute malignant colonic obstruction seems to be supported by cost-effectiveness studies and several pooled analyses that demonstrate efficacy and safety. The use of colonic stenting for palliation of patients with locally advanced or metastatic disease is much more strongly supported by retrospective and prospective studies although careful selection of the patients is paramount to avoid unexpected complications such as beavacizumab-related perforation.

REFERENCES

1. Loizou LA, Grigg D, Boulos PB, et al. Endoscopic Nd:YAG laser treatment of rectosigmoid cancer. Gut 1990;31:812–6.
2. Gevers AM, Macken E, Hiele M, et al. Endoscopic laser therapy for palliation of patients with distal colorectal carcinoma: analysis of factors influencing long-term outcome. Gastrointest Endosc 2000;51:580–5.
3. Lelcuk S, Ratan J, Klausner JM, et al. Endoscopic decompression of acute colonic obstruction. Avoiding staged surgery. Ann Surg 1986;203:292–4.
4. Dohmoto M, Rupp KD, Hohlbach G. Endoscopically-implanted prosthesis in rectal carcinoma. Dtsch Med Wochenschr 1990;115:915 [in German].
5. Spinelli P, Dal Fante M, Mancini A. Self-expanding mesh stent for endoscopic palliation of rectal obstructing tumors: a preliminary report. Surg Endosc 1992;6:72–4.
6. Tejero E, Mainar A, Fernandez L, et al. New procedure for the treatment of colorectal neoplastic obstructions. Dis Colon Rectum 1994;37:1158–9.
7. Rey JF, Romanczyk T, Greff M. Metal stents for palliation of rectal carcinoma: a preliminary report on 12 patients. Endoscopy 1995;27:501–4.
8. Fan YB, Cheng YS, Chen NW, et al. Clinical application of self-expanding metallic stent in the management of acute left-sided colorectal malignant obstruction. World J Gastroenterol 2006;12:755–9.
9. Xinopoulos D, Dimitroulopoulos D, Theodosopoulos T, et al. Stenting or stoma creation for patients with inoperable malignant colonic obstructions? Results of a study and cost-effectiveness analysis. Surg Endosc 2004;18:421–6.
10. Camúñez F, Echenagusia A, Simó G, et al. Malignant colorectal obstruction treated by means of self-expanding metallic stents: effectiveness before surgery and in palliation. Radiology 2000;216:492–7.
11. Roeland E, von Gunten CF. Current concepts in malignant bowel obstruction management. Curr Oncol Rep 2009;11:298–303.
12. Dronamraju SS, Ramamurthy S, Kelly SB, et al. Role of self-expanding metallic stents in the management of malignant obstruction of the proximal colon. Dis Colon Rectum 2009;52:1657–61.
13. Dastur JK, Forshaw MJ, Modarai B, et al. Comparison of short- and long-term outcomes following either insertion of self-expanding metallic stents or emergency surgery in malignant large bowel obstruction. Tech Coloproctol 2008;12:51–5.
14. Watt AM, Faragher IG, Griffin TT, et al. Self-expanding metallic stents for relieving malignant colorectal obstruction: a systematic review. Ann Surg 2007;246:24–30.
15. Riedl S, Wiebelt H, Bergmann U, et al. Postoperative complications and fatalities in surgical therapy of colon carcinoma: results of the German multicenter study by the Colorectal Carcinoma Study Group. Chirurg 1995;66:597–606.
16. Phillips RK, Hittinger R, Fry JS, et al. Malignant large bowel obstruction. Br J Surg 1985;72:296–302.
17. Umpleby HC, Williamson RC. Survival in acute obstructing colorectal carcinoma. Dis Colon Rectum 1984;27:299–304.

18. Mella J, Biffin A, Radcliffe AG, et al. Population-based audit of colorectal cancer management in two UK health regions. Br J Surg 1997;84:1731–6.
19. Serpell JW, McDermott FT, Katrivessis H, et al. Obstructing carcinomas of the colon. Br J Surg 1989;76:965–9.
20. Zorcolo L, Covotta L, Carlomagno N, et al. Safety of primary anastomosis in emergency colo-rectal surgery. Colorectal Disease 2003;5:262–9.
21. Villar JM, Martinez AP, Villegas MT, et al. Surgical options for malignant left-sided colonic obstruction. Surg Today 2005;35:275–81.
22. Biondo S, Pares D, Frago R, et al. Large bowel obstruction: predictive factors for postoperative mortality. Dis Colon Rectum 2004;47(11):1889–97.
23. Hsu TC. Comparison of one-stage resection and anastomosis of acute complete obstruction of left and right colon. Am J Surg 2005;189:384–7.
24. Goyal A, Schein M. Current practices in left-sided colonic emergencies. A survey of US gastrointestinal surgeons. Dig Surg 2001;18:399–402.
25. Zorcolo L, Covotta L, Carlomagno N, et al. Toward lowering morbidity, mortality and stoma formation in emergency colorectal surgery: the role of specialization. Dis Colon Rectum 2003;46:1461–8.
26. Tekkis PP, Kinsman R, Thompson MR, et al. The Association of Coloproctology of Great Britain and Ireland study of large bowel obstruction caused by colorectal cancer. Ann Surg 2004;204:76–81.
27. Darby CR, Berry AR, Mortensen N. Management variability in surgery for colo-rectal emergencies. Br J Surg 1992;79:206–10.
28. Trompetas V. Emergency management of malignant acute left sided colonic obstruction. Ann R Coll Surg Engl 2008;90:181–6.
29. Baron TH. Colonic stenting: technique, technology, and outcomes for malignant and benign disease. Gastrointest Endosc Clin N Am 2005;15:757–71.
30. Keswani RN, Azar RR, Edmundowicz SA, et al. Stenting for malignant colonic obstruction: a comparison of efficacy and complications in colonic versus extracolonic malignancy. Gastrointest Endosc 2009;69:675–80.
31. Trompetas V, Saunders M, Gossage J, et al. Shortcomings in colonic stenting to palliate large bowel obstruction from extracolonic malignancies. Int J Colorectal Dis 2010;25:851–4.
32. Tack J, Gevers AM, Rutgeerts P. Self-expandable metallic stents in the palliation of rectosigmoidal carcinoma: a follow-up study. Gastrointest Endosc 1998;48:267–71.
33. Shellock FG, Crues JV. MR procedures: biologic effects, safety, and patient care. Radiology 2004;232:635–52.
34. Nitatori T, Hanaoka H, Hachiya J, et al. MRI artifacts of metallic stents derived from imaging sequencing and the ferromagnetic nature of materials. Radiat Med 1999;17:329–34.
35. Taal BG, Muller SH, Boot H, et al. Potential risks and artifacts of magnetic resonance imaging of self-expandable esophageal stents. Gastrointest Endosc 1997;46:424–9.
36. Cha EY, Park SH, Lee SS. CT colonography after metallic stent placement for acute malignant colonic obstruction. Radiology 2010;254:774–82.
37. Bielawska B, Hookey LC, Jalink D. Large-diameter self-expanding metal stents appear to be safe and effective for malignant colonic obstruction with and without concurrent use of chemotherapy. Surg Endosc 2010;24:2814–21.
38. Sebastian S, Johnston S, Geoghegan T, et al. Pooled analysis of the efficacy and safety of self-expanding metal stenting in malignant colorectal obstruction. Am J Gastroenterol 2004;99:2051–7.

39. Choi JS, Choo SW, Park KB, et al. Interventional management of malignant colorectal obstruction: use of covered and uncovered stents. Korean J Radiol 2007;8: 57–63.
40. Park S, Cheon JH, Park JJ, et al. Comparison of efficacies between stents for malignant colorectal obstruction: a randomized prospective study. Gastrointest Endosc 2010;71:304–10.
41. Choo IW, Do YS, Suh SW, et al. Malignant colorectal obstruction: treatment with a flexible covered stent. Radiology 1998;206:415–21.
42. Lee KM, Shin SJ, Hwang JC, et al. Comparison of uncovered stent with covered stent for treatment of malignant colorectal obstruction. Gastrointest Endosc 2007; 66:931–6.
43. Baron TH, Dean PA, Yates MD 3rd, et al. Expandable metal stent for colonic obstruction: techniques and outcome. Gastrointest Endosc 1998;47:277–86.
44. Small AJ, Coelho-Prabhu N, Baron TH. Endoscopic placement of self-expandable metal stents for malignant colonic obstruction: longterm outcomes and complication factors. Gastrointest Endosc 2010;71:560–72.
45. Tanaka A, Sadahiro S, Yasuda M, et al. Endoscopic balloon dilation for obstructive colorectal cancer: a basic study on morphologic and pathologic features associated with perforation. Gastrointest Endosc 2010;71:799–805.
46. Vázquez-Iglesias JL, Gonzalez-Conde B, Vázquez-Millán MA, et al. Self-expandable stents in malignant colonic obstruction: insertion assisted with a sphincterotome in technically difficult cases. Gastrointest Endosc 2005;62:436–7.
47. Cennamo V, Fuccio L, Laterza L, et al. Side-viewing endoscope for colonic self-expandable metal stenting in patients with malignant colonic obstruction. Eur J Gastroenterol Hepatol 2009;21:585–6.
48. Baron TH. Indications and results of endoscopic rectal stenting. J Gastrointest Surg 2004;8:266–9.
49. García-Cano J, González-Huix F, Juzgao D, et al. Use of self-expanding metal stents to treat malignant colorectal obstruction in general endoscopic practice. Gastrointest Endosc 2006;64:914–20.
50. Kim JS, Hur H, Min BS, et al. Oncologic outcomes of self-expanding metallic stent insertion as a bridge to surgery in the management of left-sided colon cancer obstruction: comparison with non-obstructing elective surgery. World J Surg 2009;33:1281–6.
51. Kleespies A, Fuessl KE, Seeliger H, et al. Determinants of morbidity and survival after elective non-curative resection of stage IV colon and rectal cancer. Int J Colorectal Dis 2009;24:1097–109.
52. Hotokezaka M, Jimi S, Hidaka H, et al. Factors influencing outcome after surgery for stage IV colorectal cancer. Surg Today 2008;38:784–9.
53. Ratto C, Sofo L, Ippoliti M, et al. Prognostic factors in colorectal cancer. Literature review for clinical application. Dis Colon Rectum 1998;41:1033–49.
54. Katoh H, Yamashita K, Kokuba Y, et al. Surgical resection of stage IV colorectal cancer and prognosis. World J Surg 2008;32:1130–7.
55. Fiori E, Lamazza A, De Cesare A, et al. Palliative management of malignant rectosigmoidal obstruction. Colostomy vs. endoscopic stenting. A randomized prospective trial. Anticancer Res 2004;24:265–8.
56. van Hooft JE, Fockens P, Marinelli AW, et al, Dutch Colorectal Stent Group. Early closure of a multicenter randomized clinical trial of endoscopic stenting versus surgery for stage IV left sided colorectal cancer. Endoscopy 2008;40:184–91.
57. van Hooft JE, Fockens P, Marinelli AW, et al, On behalf of the Dutch Stent-in I study group. Premature closure of the Dutch Stent-in I study. Lancet 2006;368:1573–4.

58. Repici A, De Caro G, Luigiano C, et al. WallFlex colonic stent placement for management of malignant colonic obstruction: a prospective study at two centers. Gastrointest Endosc 2008;67:77–84.

59. Brehant O, Fuks D, Bartoli E, et al. Bridge to surgery stenting in patients with malignant colonic obstruction using the WallFlex colonic stent: report of a prospective multicenter registry. Colorectal Disease 2009;11:178–83.

60. Repici A, Adler DG, Gibbs CM, et al. Stenting of the proximal colon in patients with malignant large bowel obstruction: techniques and outcomes. Gastrointest Endosc 2007;66:940–4.

61. Baraza W, Lee F, Brown S, et al. Combination endo-radiological colorectal stenting: a prospective 5-year clinical evaluation. Colorectal Dis 2008;10:901–6.

62. Law WL, Choi HK, Chu KW. Comparison of stenting with emergency surgery as palliative treatment for obstructing primary left-sided colorectal cancer. Br J Surg 2003;90:1429–33.

63. Im JP, Kim SG, Kang HW, et al. Clinical outcomes and patency of self-expanding metal stents in patients with malignant colorectal obstruction: a prospective single center study. Int J Colorectal Dis 2008;23:789–94.

64. Repici A, Fregonese D, Costamagna G, et al. Ultraflex precision colonic stent placement for palliation of malignant colonic obstruction: a prospective multicenter study. Gastrointest Endosc 2007;66:920–7.

65. Karoui M, Charachon A, Delbaldo C, et al. Stents for palliation of obstructive metastatic colon cancer: impact on management and chemotherapy administration. Arch Surg 2007;142:619–23.

66. Faragher IG, Chaitowitz IM, Stupart DA. Long-term results of palliative stenting or surgery for incurable obstructing colon cancer. Colorectal Dis 2008;10:668–72.

67. Small AJ, Baron TH. Comparison of Wallstent and Ultraflex stents for palliation of malignant left-sided colon obstruction: a retrospective, case-matched analysis. Gastrointest Endosc 2008;67:478–88.

68. Vemulapalli R, Lara LF, Sreenarasimhaiah J, et al. A comparison of palliative stenting or emergent surgery for obstructing incurable colon cancer. Dig Dis Sci 2010;55:1732–7.

69. Jung MK, Park SY, Jeon SW. Factors associated with the long-term outcome of a self-expandable colon stent used for palliation of malignant colorectal obstruction. Surg Endosc 2010;24:525–30.

70. Manes G, de Bellis M, Fuccio L, et al. Endoscopic palliation of patients with incurable malignant colorectal obstruction by means of a self expanding metal stent. Analysis of results and predictors of outcome in a large multicenter series. Arch Surg, in press.

71. Lee HJ, Hong SP, Cheon JH, et al. Long-term outcome of palliative therapy for malignant colorectal obstruction in patients with unresectable metastatic colorectal cancers: endoscopic stenting versus surgery. Gastrointest Endosc 2011;73(3):535–42.

72. Varadarajulu S, Roy A, Lopes T, et al. Endoscopic stenting versus surgical colostomy for the management of malignant colonic obstruction: comparison of hospital costs and clinical outcomes. Surg Endosc 2011. [Epub ahead of print].

73. Nagula S, Ishill N, Nash C, et al. Quality of life and symptom control after stent placement or surgical palliation of malignant colorectal obstruction. J Am Coll Surg 2010;210:45–53.

74. Morino M, Bertello A, Garbarini A, et al. Malignant colonic obstruction managed by endoscopic stent decompression followed by laparoscopic resections. Surg Endosc 2002;16:1483–7.

75. Stipa F, Pigazzi A, Bascone B, et al. Management of obstructive colorectal cancer with endoscopic stenting followed by single-stage surgery: open or laparoscopic resection? Surg Endosc 2008;22:1477–81.

76. Olmi S, Scaini A, Cesana G, et al. Acute colonic obstruction: endoscopic stenting and laparascopic resection. Surg Endosc 2007;21:2100–4.

77. Martinez-Santos C, Lobato RF, Fradejas JM, et al. Self-expandable stent before elective surgery vs. emergency surgery for the treatment of malignant colorectal obstruction: comparison of primary anastomosis and morbidity rates. Dis Colon Rectum 2002;45:401–6.

78. Repici A, Conio M, Caronna S, et al. Early and late outcomes of patients with obstructing colorectal cancer treated by stenting and elective surgery: a comparison with emergency surgery and patients operated without obstructive symptoms. Gastrointest Endosc 2004;59:AB275.

79. Breitenstein S, Rickenbacher A, Berdajs D, et al. Systematic evaluation of surgical strategies for acute malignant left-sided colonic obstruction. Br J Surg 2007;94:1451–60.

80. Cheung HY, Chung CC, Tsang WW, et al. Endolaparoscopic approach vs conventional open surgery in the treatment of obstructing left-sided colon cancer: a randomized controlled trial. Arch Surg 2009;144:1127–32.

81. Pirlet IA, Slim K, Kwiatkowski F, et al. Emergency preoperative stenting versus surgery for acute left-sided malignant colonic obstruction: a multicenter randomized controlled trial. Surg Endosc 2010. [Epub ahead of print].

82. van Hooft Je, Bemelan WA, Oldenburg B, et al. Colonic stenting versus emergency surgery for acute left-sided malignant colonic obstruction a multicentre randomised study. Lancet Oncol 2011;12(4):344–52.

83. Maruthachalam K, Lash GE, Shenton BK, et al. Tumour cell dissemination following endoscopic stent insertion. Br J Surg 2007;94:1151–4.

84. Saida Y, Sumiyama Y, Nagao J, et al. Long-term prognosis of preoperative 'bridge to surgery' expandable metallic stent insertion for obstructive colorectal cancer: comparison with emergency operation. Dis Colon Rectum 2003; 46(Suppl):S44–9.

85. Targownik LE, Spiegel BM, Sack J, et al. Colonic stent vs. emergency surgery for management of acute left-sided malignant colonic obstruction: a decision analysis. Gastrointest Endosc 2004;60:865–74.

86. Singh H, Latosinsky S, Spiegel BM, et al. The cost-effectiveness of colonic stenting as a bridge to curative surgery in patients with acute left-sided malignant colonic obstruction: a Canadian perspective. Can J Gastroenterol 2006;20: 779–85.

87. Osman HS, Rashid HI, Sathananthan N, et al. The cost effectiveness of self-expanding metal stents in the management of malignant left-sided large bowel obstruction. Colorectal Dis 2000;2:233–7.

88. Binkert CA, Ledermann H, Jost R, et al. Acute colonic obstruction: clinical aspects and cost-effectiveness of preoperative and palliative treatment with self-expanding metallic stents–a preliminary report. Radiology 1998;206:199–204.

89. Khot UP, Lang AW, Murali K, et al. Systemic review of the efficacy of colorectal stents. Br J Surg 2002;89:1096–102.

90. Suh JP, Kim SW, Cho YK, et al. Effectiveness of stent placement for palliative treatment in malignant colorectal obstruction and predictive factors for stent occlusion. Surg Endosc 2010;24:400–6.

91. Baron TH. Minimizing endoscopic complications: endoluminal stents. Gastrointest Endosc Clin N Am 2007;17:83–104.

92. Dharmadhikari R, Nice C. Complications of colonic stenting: a pictorial review. Abdom Imaging 2008;33:278–84.

93. Alcantara M, Serra X, Bombardo J, et al. Colorectal stenting as an effective therapy for preoperative and palliative treatment of large bowel obstruction: 9 years' experience. Tech Coloproctol 2007;11:316–22.

94. Datye A, Hersh J. Colonic perforation after stent placement for malignant colorectal obstruction - causes and contributing factors. Minim Invasive Ther Allied Technol 2010. [Epub ahead of print].

95. Cennamo V, Fuccio L, Mutri V, et al. Does stent placement for advanced colon cancer increase the risk of perforation during bevacizumab-based therapy? Clin Gastroenterol Hepatol 2009;7:1174–6.

96. Hapani S, Chu D, Wu S. Risk of gastrointestinal perforation in patients with cancer treated with bevacizumab: a meta-analysis. Lancet Oncol 2009;10:559–68.

Expandable Stents: Unique Devices and Clinical Uses

Andrew S. Ross, MD*, Richard A. Kozarek, MD

KEYWORDS

- Expandable stents • Gastroenterology • Endoscopy
- Endoprostheses

For more than a century, stents have been used for a variety of clinical indications, both benign and malignant, in the gastrointestinal (GI) tract. The principle is rather simple: an occluded lumen is bypassed by the placement of a prosthesis, essentially creating a new pathway for the flow of food, stool, bile, and pancreatic juice. Although the basic premise behind stenting within the GI tract has not changed over time, the stents themselves have.[1]

For example, the earliest stents used within the esophagus were fashioned from ivory and sandalwood. In the 1970s, small-diameter, rigid, plastic stents requiring pre-assembly were used within the esophagus. The past 40 years have witnessed the progression from these devices to self-expanding stents made from various metals and plastics. Self-expanding metal stents (SEMS) for use in the esophagus are now available in both partially and fully covered versions.[1]

Technological modifications in stent design have not been limited to the esophagus nor have they been limited to SEMS. Stents designed for the pancreaticobiliary tree, colon, and duodenum have all witnessed changes over the past 40 years. Plastic stents are now available in straight, single, and double pigtail versions. These changes in stent technology along with changes in endoscopy have opened the door for novel (and off-label) uses of these devices throughout the GI tract. This article attempts to characterize some of the novel and unique uses of endoprostheses, both plastic and SEMS as well as self-expanding plastic stents (SEPS), throughout the GI tract.

BARIATRIC SURGERY

The obesity epidemic throughout North America has resulted in increased performance of bariatric surgery. The most common operation performed is the roux-en-Y gastric bypass (RYGB). Although high rates of success have been seen in terms of loss of

Digestive Disease Institute, Virginia Mason Medical Center, Mailstop C3-GAS, 1100 9th Avenue, Seattle, WA 98101, USA
* Corresponding author.
E-mail address: andrew.ross@vmmc.org

Gastrointest Endoscopy Clin N Am 21 (2011) 535–545
doi:10.1016/j.giec.2011.04.003
1052-5157/11/$ – see front matter © 2011 Elsevier Inc. All rights reserved.

excess weight and resolution of diabetes, operative complications can occur in up to 9% of patients.[2–5] Anastamotic leaks at the gastrojejunostomy are one such complication (**Fig. 1**) and recent reports suggest significant rates of successful treatment following the placement of covered SEMS or SEPS. In one of the largest series to date, Eubanks and colleagues[3] reported an 84% rate of leak closure in 19 patients who had undergone placement of a covered SEMS or SEPS for the treatment anastamotic leaks following RYGB. In addition, immediate symptomatic improvement occurred in 90% of the treated patients and 79% had oral feeding initiated once the stent had been placed. Stent migration occurred in 58% of the stents placed with 3 patients requiring surgical removal for migration into the small intestine.

Stent placement for managing anastamotic leaks following RYGB is straightforward. Because of the postsurgical nature of the intestine at the time of endoscopy, the most significant challenge tends to be identifying the gastrojejunostomy and Roux limb. Because the leaks can be significant, it is common to visualize the peritoneal cavity at the time of endoscopy (see **Fig. 1**). Once the Roux limb has been entered, however, marking the distal margin of anticipated stent placement with either submucosal contrast injection or hemoclip placement is performed. A wire guide can then be left in place and the stent deployed in the usual fashion under fluoroscopic and, in some cases, endoscopic control. If fluoroscopy alone is used the proximal aspect of anticipated stent placement, typically within the mid to distal esophagus to anchor and potentially minimize risk of migration, should be marked as well. The authors select the largest caliber stent available to decrease the risk of stent migration. An upper GI series can be performed immediately following stent placement to confirm that the leak has been sealed and, if so, the stent is left in place for 6 weeks (**Fig. 2**). Migrated stents can be retrieved endoscopically or, if unsuccessful, surgically.

In patients who have developed chronic fistula the duration of stent placement may be considerably longer (up to months) and may require adjuvant therapy, such as application of tissue adhesives.

LUMINAL RECONSTITUTION

SEPS and covered SEMS have been used in luminal reconstitution, both in the colon and esophagus. On occasion, patients who have undergone segmental colonic

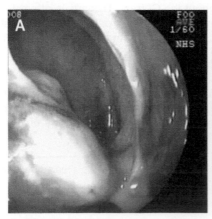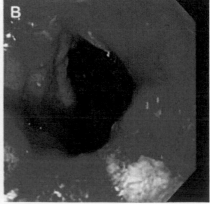

Fig. 1. (*A*) Endoscopic appearance of the gastrojejunostomy immediately following Roux-en-Y gastric bypass demonstrating a large leak; the peritoneal cavity is readily visible. (*B*) The same anastamosis following 6 weeks of stenting with a fully covered esophageal stent.

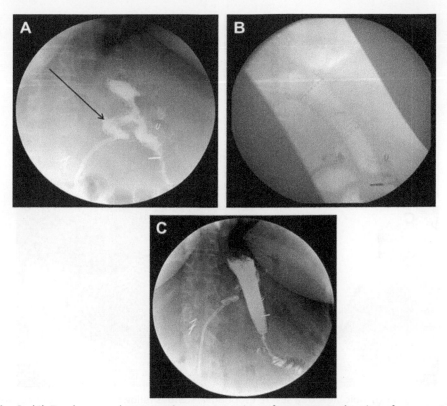

Fig. 2. (*A*) Esophagram demonstrating extravasation of contrast at the site of an anasta-motic leak (*arrow*) following Roux-en-Y gastric bypass. (*B*) A SEPS is placed across the site of leak. (*C*) Esophagram following SEPS placement demonstrating resolution of the leak.

resection can present with complete obstruction of the surgical anastamosis. This presentation is likely caused by chronic inflammation and scarring at the anastamo-sis, poor surgical technique, or regional ischemia. Similarly, patients with a history of caustic ingestion, mediastinal radiation, or desquamating inflammatory processes of the esophagus may present with a complete esophageal obstruction (**Fig. 3**). Although a complete postsurgical colonic anastamotic obstruction can be easily treated with a diverting ileostomy, a complete esophageal obstruction presents a greater clinical challenge and may require esophagectomy, colonic interposition, or the creation of a spit fistula and feeding via a gastrostomy.

Several reports have appeared in the literature describing bidirectional endoscopy, either through the ileostomy and rectum (**Figs. 4** and **5**) or mouth and through a gas-trostomy tract (see **Fig. 3**), with subsequent luminal recanalization.[6] Much like the placement of an endoscopic gastrostomy, the endoscopes are brought within milli-meters of each other at the site of stenosis. In most cases, transillumination through the stenosis can be recognized and an endoscopic ultrasound needle is passed through the bowel wall under direct endoscopic and fluoroscopic control. A wire can then be passed through the needle and grasped using a snare passed through the second endoscope. Placement of double pigtail stents through the newly formed lumen can then be performed followed weeks later by the placement of a SEPS or

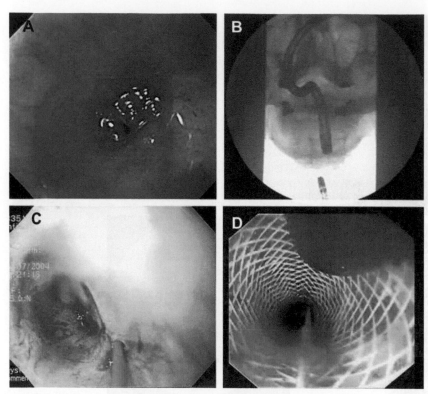

Fig. 3. (*A*) Endoscopic view of a severe esophageal stenosis following radiation therapy for a head and neck cancer. (*B*) Endoscopes are passed per os and via an existing gastrostomy and a wire guide is passed through the stenosis in a retrograde fashion (*C*). (*D*) A fully covered SEPS is placed across the stenosis completing the luminal reconstitution.

covered SEMS. Pneumoperitoneum or pneumomediastinum can be seen (see **Fig. 4**) following luminal recanalization, although peritonitis and mediastinitis typically do not occur.

DRAINAGE OF THE BILIARY TREE

Although endoscopic retrograde cholangiopancreatography has made access to and drainage of the biliary tract through the major papilla a straightforward undertaking, access failure occurs in up to 10% of patients with native pancreaticobiliary anatomy. In such patients, the standard approach in most centers is to refer patients to interventional radiology for percutaneous drainage of the biliary tree. Percutaneous biliary drains are not without their own set of complications, including bleeding, bile leak, infection, and tube occlusion requiring reintervention. In addition, patient discomfort from drain placement either through the abdominal wall or intercostal space cannot be minimized.

With the evolution of endoscopic ultrasound (EUS) from a purely diagnostic tool into a therapeutic modality, strictures or collections within close proximity to the esophagus, stomach, duodenum, and (sometimes) rectum have become targets for EUS-directed therapeutic interventions. Regarding the biliary tree in particular, EUS-guided rendezvous has been reported in cases where retrograde access to the biliary tree has failed

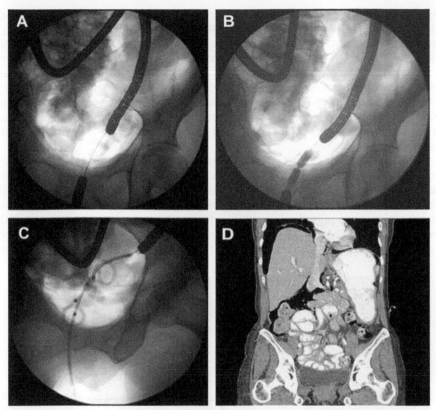

Fig. 4. (*A*) Fluoroscopic view of a rendezvous luminal reconstitution in the rectosigmoid; wire-guide access is obtained across a complete anastamotic stenosis. Balloon dilation is then performed (*B*) and plastic double pigtail stents are placed (*C*). Asymptomatic pneumoperitoneum was seen following the procedure (*D*).

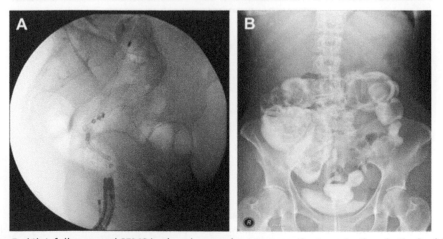

Fig. 5. (*A*) A fully covered SEMS is placed across the anastamotic stenosis; the plastic double pigtail stents are removed. (*B*) Barium enema demonstrating a patent anastamosis following luminal reconstitution using a SEMS.

or is not technically feasible.[7–9] Working through the stomach, a fine-needle aspiration (FNA) needle can be directed into a dilated biliary tree in the left lobe of the liver (**Fig. 6**). A dilated common bile duct can also be accessed through the duodenum. A wire can then be advanced through the needle into the biliary tree and directed toward the duodenum, crossing the papilla in an antegrade fashion. If the papilla can be crossed, the echoendoscope is withdrawn and replaced with a duodenoscope, which can then be used to complete the procedure in a rendezvous fashion. In some cases, however, the bile papilla cannot be crossed by the wire guide in an antegrade fashion or the papilla is not accessible endoscopically, such as occurs with a severe stenosis or gastric outlet obstruction, respectively.

In cases where rendezvous access is not possible, stents can be used to create a choledochoduodenostomy or choledochogastrostomy effectively allowing the biliary tree to drain directly into the stomach or duodenum.[7–9] Straight and pigtail plastic stents as well as covered and uncovered SEMS have been used in this setting. The technique is straightforward; access to the biliary tree is obtained under EUS control and a guidewire is left in place. Next, a tract is created using a needle knife or dilating catheter. Dilation of the tract, typically through the use of a graduated

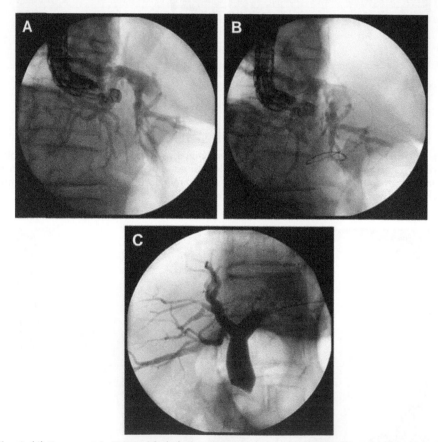

Fig. 6. (A) Transgastric EUS-guided cholangiogram demonstrating a dilated biliary tree in a patient with a duodenal carcinoma. (B) Wire-guide access is obtained. (C) A 5Fr cannula is advanced through the tract to the level of the stenosis in an attempt to achieve transpapillary access.

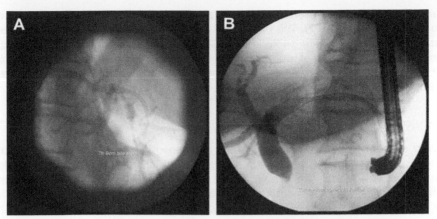

Fig. 7. (*A*) Transgastric placement of a plastic bile duct stent into the biliary tree in the left lobe of the liver. (*B*) Transgastric placement of a fully covered SEMS into the biliary tree in the left lobe of the liver.

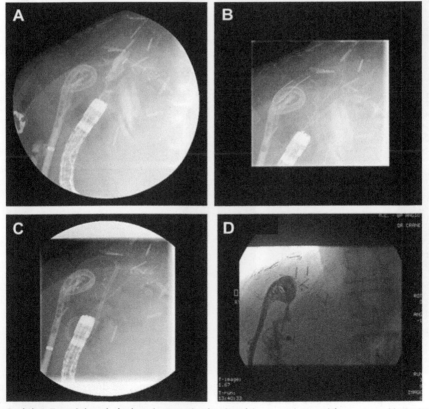

Fig. 8. (*A*) A Transjejunal cholangiogram is obtained in a patient with roux-en-Y anatomy and a drained bile leak following a trisegmentectomy for cholangiocarcinoma. A wire guide is passed into the opacified bile duct (*B*) and a plastic double pigtail stent is placed (*C*). A radiographic drain study (*D*) demonstrates free flow of contrast into the jejunum, allowing the percutaneous drain to be eventually removed.

dilating catheter, is then performed so that a stent of the requisite size can be passed into the biliary tree (**Fig. 7**). The biliary tree can also be drained by transenteric stent placement in patients with postsurgical biliary anatomy (**Fig. 8**). Like percutaneous biliary drainage, the major complications of this approach are bleeding and bile leak, pneumoperitoneum can also be seen. The risk of bile leak is partially mitigated by approaching the biliary tree through the left lobe of the liver.

DRAINAGE OF THE PANCREAS

Walled-off pancreatic necrosis (WOPN) is often seen in the setting of severe acute pancreatitis where devitalized pancreatic tissue and fluid organizes into a collection that may act as a nidus for infection. Left untreated, infected WOPN is associated with a mortality rate that reaches close to 100%. The historical gold standard for the treatment of infected WOPN has been surgical necrosectomy, however, the

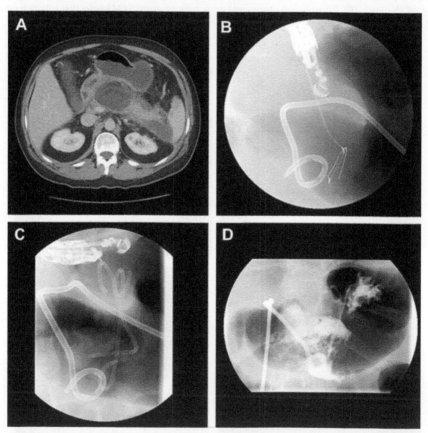

Fig. 9. (A) Severe pancreatic necrosis and a resultant disconnected duct. Following percutaneous drain placement, EUS-guided access is obtained to the necroma (B) allowing placement of 2 double pigtail plastic stents (C). Injection of contrast through the percutaneous drain (D) demonstrates free flow of contrast into the stomach through the newly created internal fistula. This procedure will allow eventual removal of the percutaneous drainage catheter once the necroma has resolved; a chronic pancreaticocutaneous fistula will likely be avoided in this case because of the transgastric drains.

high associated operative morbidity and significant mortality rates seen with this operation have spawned investigation into less invasive means of debridement. Multiple descriptions are now seen in the literature on minimally invasive approaches to pancreatic debridement, including laparoscopic, nephroscopic, endoscopic, and percutaneous, as well as combined endoscopic and percutaneous.[10–16]

Stents, both SEMS and plastic, play an important role in endoscopic and sometimes percutaneous approaches to debridement of infected WOPN. When the necroma is located within close proximity (<2 cm) of the gastric or duodenal wall, endoscopic access can typically be obtained with or without the use of endoscopic ultrasound (see **Fig. 8**). Debridement is then performed using a variety of endoscopic accessories.[12] Access is then maintained between the necroma and the GI tract by the placement of either multiple double pigtail plastic stents or a covered SEMS so that the necroma can be reentered for additional debridement. In patients with the disconnected duct syndrome who undergo percutaneous drainage, the creation of a necrogastrostomy or necroduodenostomy may serve to avoid the creation of pancreaticocutaneous fistulae by diverting pancreatic juice from the disconnected portion of the gland into the stomach or duodenum (**Fig. 9**).[13]

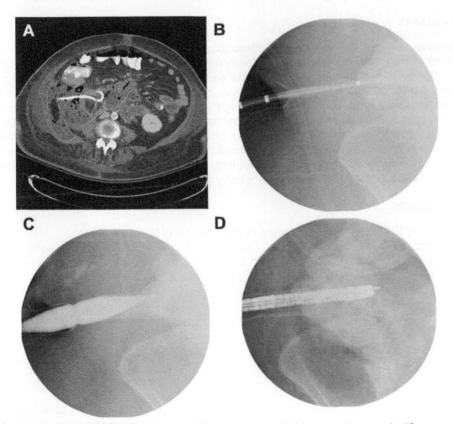

Fig. 10. (*A*) A percutaneous drainage catheter in an area of pancreatic necrosis. The necroma is located far from the gastric and duodenal wall. (*B*) A fully covered metal esophageal stent is placed through the drainage tract and is dilated (*C*) to allow passage of the endoscope (*D*), essentially acting as a conduit for endoscopic necrosectomy. (*Courtesy of* Dr Todd Baron, Rochester, MN.)

On occasion, infected WOPN may be located at some distance from the gastric or duodenal wall making endoscopic access impossible. Such cases are typically handled surgically, either open or laparoscopic, or via a percutaneous approach. Covered SEMS placement across percutaneous drainage tracts to allow for endoscopic access for debridement (**Fig. 10**) has been performed. The SEMS are used as a conduit for the endoscope, which can be removed once the debridement has been performed.

In patients with obstruction of the pancreatic duct caused by a calculus or severe stenosis, stents can be placed through the stomach directly into the pancreatic duct to create a pancreaticogastrostomy with resultant drainage of pancreatic juice into the stomach.[17] Typically, this procedure is performed as a rescue technique once attempts at obtaining retrograde access to pancreatic duct have failed. The dorsal pancreatic duct is accessed with an endosonographically directed 19-guage FNA needle. A guidewire is then passed through the needle into the pancreatic duct and an attempt at antegrade access into the duodenum is made. If this fails, the tract can be dilated using a needle knife, graduated dilating catheter, or Sohendra stent extractor subsequent to which a straight or single pigtail pancreatic stent can be placed through the gastric wall into the duct to achieve transgastric drainage.

SUMMARY

The use of stents throughout the GI tract has evolved over the past century moving away from a device used only to create new passages through obstructed ducts and lumen to one that achieves drainage and allows for endoscopic access through means that not long ago could only be imagined. The evolution of EUS from a purely diagnostic to therapeutic tool as well as significant improvements in stent design have been key factors that have allowed endoscopists to drive the use of stents in gastroenterology into a variety of new directions. Endoscopic creativity remains crucial in the evolution of any new endoscopic technology. Finally, the use of multidisciplinary teams, including endoscopists, radiologists, and surgeons, allows for the exchange of ideas and procedural planning necessary for successful innovation.

REFERENCES

1. Kang SG. Gastrointestinal stent update. Gut Liver 2010;4:S19–24.
2. Babor R, Talbot M, Tyndal A. Treatment of upper gastrointestinal leaks with a removable, covered, self-expanding metallic stent. Surg Laparosc Endosc Percutan Tech 2009;19:e1–4.
3. Eubanks S, Edwards CA, Fearing NM, et al. Use of endoscopic stents to treat anastomotic complications after bariatric surgery. J Am Coll Surg 2008;206: 935–8 [discussion: 938–9].
4. Fukumoto R, Orlina J, McGinty J, et al. Use of Polyflex stents in treatment of acute esophageal and gastric leaks after bariatric surgery. Surg Obes Relat Dis 2007;3: 68–71 [discussion: 71–2].
5. Zisis C, Guillin A, Heyries L, et al. Stent placement in the management of oesophageal leaks. Eur J Cardiothorac Surg 2008;33:451–6.
6. Maple JT, Petersen BT, Baron TH, et al. Endoscopic management of radiation-induced complete upper esophageal obstruction with an antegrade-retrograde rendezvous technique. Gastrointest Endosc 2006;64:822–8.
7. Kim YS, Gupta K, Mallery S, et al. Endoscopic ultrasound rendezvous for bile duct access using a transduodenal approach: cumulative experience at a single center. A case series. Endoscopy 2010;42:496–502.

8. Yamao K, Bhatia V, Mizuno N, et al. Interventional endoscopic ultrasonography. J Gastroenterol Hepatol 2009;24:509–19.
9. Yamao K, Hara K, Mizuno N, et al. EUS-Guided Biliary Drainage. Gut Liver 2010; 4:S67–75.
10. Freeny PC, Hauptmann E, Althaus SJ, et al. Percutaneous CT-guided catheter drainage of infected acute necrotizing pancreatitis: techniques and results. AJR Am J Roentgenol 1998;170:969–75.
11. Seewald S, Groth S, Omar S, et al. Aggressive endoscopic therapy for pancreatic necrosis and pancreatic abscess: a new safe and effective treatment algorithm (videos). Gastrointest Endosc 2005;62:92–100.
12. Seifert H, Biermer M, Schmitt W, et al. Transluminal endoscopic necrosectomy after acute pancreatitis: a multicentre study with long-term follow-up (the GEPARD Study). Gut 2009;58:1260–6.
13. Ross A, Gluck M, Irani S, et al. Combined endoscopic and percutaneous drainage of organized pancreatic necrosis. Gastrointest Endosc 2010;71:79–84.
14. van Baal MC, van Santvoort HC, Bollen TL, et al. Systematic review of percutaneous catheter drainage as primary treatment for necrotizing pancreatitis. Br J Surg 2010;98:18–27.
15. van Santvoort HC, Besselink MG, Bakker OJ, et al. A step-up approach or open necrosectomy for necrotizing pancreatitis. N Engl J Med 2010;362:1491–502.
16. Raraty MG, Halloran CM, Dodd S, et al. Minimal access retroperitoneal pancreatic necrosectomy: improvement in morbidity and mortality with a less invasive approach. Ann Surg 2010;251:787–93.
17. Shami VM, Kahaleh M. Endoscopic ultrasonography (EUS)-guided access and therapy of pancreatico-biliary disorders: EUS-guided cholangio and pancreatic drainage. Gastrointest Endosc Clin N Am 2007;17:581–93, vii–viii.

Index

Note: Page numbers of article titles are in **boldface** type.

Gastrointest Endoscopy Clin N Am 21 (2011) 547–553
doi:10.1016/S1052-5157(11)00054-7
1052-5157/11/$ – see front matter © 2011 Elsevier Inc. All rights reserved.

Moving?

Make sure your subscription moves with you!

To notify us of your new address, find your **Clinics Account Number** (located on your mailing label above your name), and contact customer service at:

Email: journalscustomerservice-usa@elsevier.com

800-654-2452 (subscribers in the U.S. & Canada)
314-447-8871 (subscribers outside of the U.S. & Canada)

Fax number: 314-447-8029

Elsevier Health Sciences Division
Subscription Customer Service
3251 Riverport Lane
Maryland Heights, MO 63043

*To ensure uninterrupted delivery of your subscription, please notify us at least 4 weeks in advance of move.